SLIMMING
The Complete Guide

New revised edition

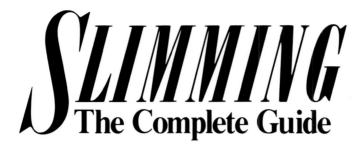

SLIMMING
The Complete Guide

By the Experts of Slimming Magazine

Introduction by Audrey Eyton

New revised edition

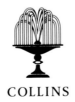

COLLINS

For all the recipes in this book, quantities are given
in both metric and imperial measures. These are not
exact conversions. Follow either set but not a mixture
of both because they are not interchangeable. If you are
dieting by counting kilojoules rather than calories, use
the conversion rate 1 calorie = 4.2 kilojoules.

Slimming magazine contributors:

Editor: Sybil Greatbatch
Nutritionist: Dr Elizabeth Evans
Home economist: Glynis McGuinness
Contributing editor: Gaynor Hagan
Consultant: Patience Bulkeley, Editor of Slimming
  Magazine

William Collins Sons & Co Ltd
London · Glasgow · Sydney
Auckland · Toronto · Johannesburg

First published in 1982
Reprinted 1982, 1983, 1984
New revised edition 1987

First edition designed by Sackville Design Group Ltd
78 Margaret Street, London W1N 7HB

British Library Cataloguing in Publication Data

Slimming: the complete guide.—New rev. ed.
  1. Reducing
  I. Slimming Magazine
  613.2'5   RM222.2

  ISBN 0–00–412223–2
  ISBN 0–00–412222–4 Pbk

Printed and bound in Great Britain by
William Collins Sons & Co Ltd, Glasgow

Contents

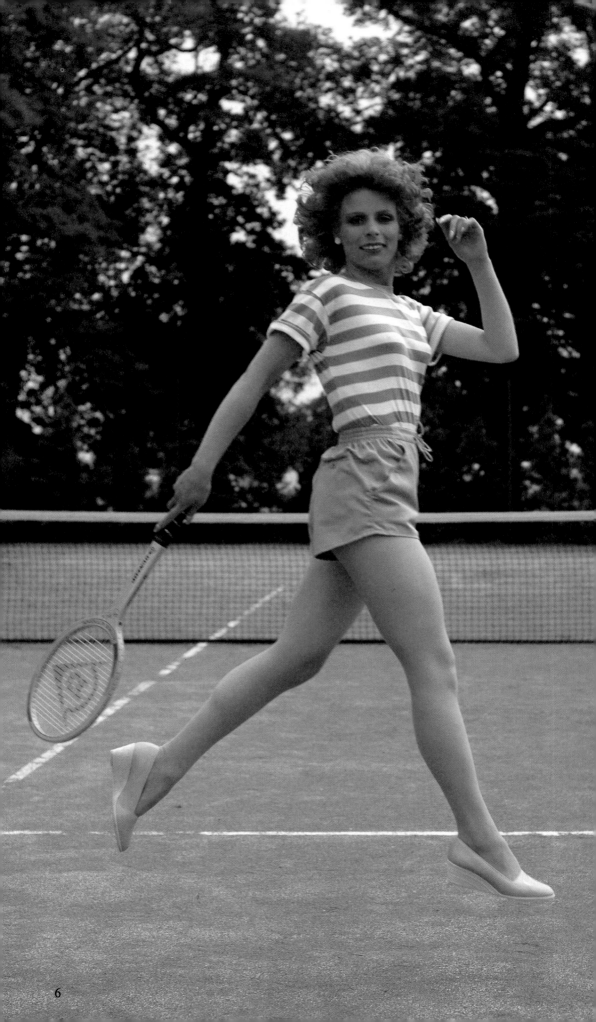

Introduction

by Audrey Eyton,
**founder-editor of Slimming Magazine
and now Editorial Consultant**

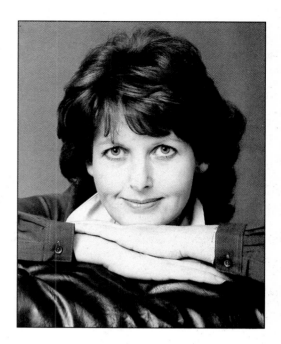

'A magazine all about slimming! But surely there isn't much to write about *that*?' Surprising as it now seems, that was the general response to the idea of a publication devoted entirely to weight problems, just before *Slimming Magazine* was launched some eighteen years ago.

Today, the fact that this entire book is devoted to that subject isn't so surprising. And very many people will warmly welcome so much helpful information on such an incredibly complex subject. Complex? Well, think of the great Western weight dilemma. In countries like Britain, at least 50 per cent of the population are a little heavier than they would like to be — if not a lot heavier. This is not a problem of mild concern, either. A large amount of surplus weight can crush self-confidence and overshadow a life, but even a small surplus can often be the cause of quite disproportionate distress.

Yet here is the odd thing. This hugely prevalent problem is one that can be solved. In 99.9 per cent of cases, overweight people can achieve their ideal weight simply by reducing their calorie consumption. But what about those infuriatingly-thin people who smugly announce: 'Weight problems? I don't know why there's so much fuss — it's just a matter of eating less, isn't it?' Well, although they may be correct on a point of fact they are utterly wrong in their lack of perception and understanding.

Eating less is not so easy. To begin with, we live in a society where practically every other television advertisement, poster, shop window, supermarket shelf, descriptive restaurant menu and strategically-placed food-dispensing machine is designed to encourage us to eat *more*. Counteracting this pressure and the many other pressures which motivate us to eat requires a great deal of self-knowledge and understanding. We need to understand why we binge and snack against our conscious will. We need to become aware of the triggers which spark off this behaviour, so that we can avoid contact with them.

But such knowledge cannot provide the complete solution to a weight problem. Who, for instance, could possibly hope to get slim and stay slim permanently without an understanding of calories? This would be like trying to learn to write without knowing the alphabet. Whether you gain or lose weight depends entirely on whether you consume more or fewer calories than your body uses up in energy.

Of course, the type of food you choose to eat will make a big difference in determining whether you are able to keep to your daily calorie quota. If, for instance, you were to choose a high proportion of fatty foods, you would get very little indeed for a weight-shedding daily allowance of 1,000 calories. One well-buttered cheese sandwich, for instance, could easily use up more than half of it. It is now universally-accepted that the type of menu which will be the most successful in helping you to lose weight will be basically low in fat and contain a high percentage of foods which give maximum filling power for minimum calories.

A menu which sufficiently reduces calorie intake and provides the foods which are most helpful and healthful is called 'a good slimming diet'. There are a number of these in this book because the eating pattern which most helps one person can prove least helpful to another.

Exercise is yet another factor in weight control. Not just one type of exercise, either (slimming is never as simple as that!). There are exercises which help you to resist weight gain, by burning up a significant quantity of calories, and there are other exercises which are practically useless in that direction, but do a splendid job in firming flabby muscles.

'Weight problems? I don't know why there's so much fuss — it's just a matter of eating less, isn't it?' What a silly oversimplification! But don't be put off by the complexity of the task. This book is full of information that will make everything clear, with the added inspiration that comes from learning how others faced the same hurdles and conquered weight problems that were every bit as complex as your own.

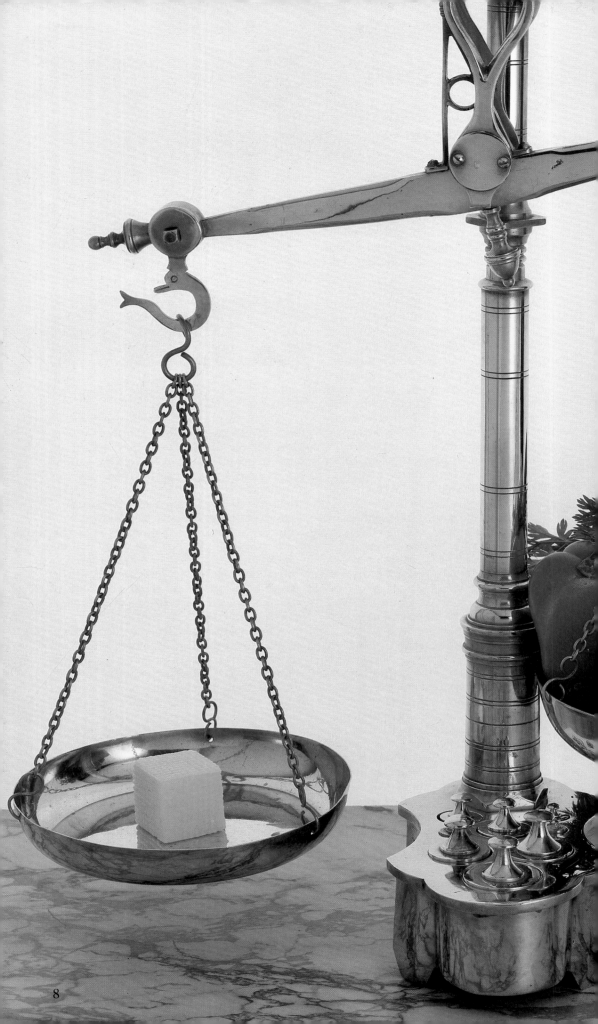

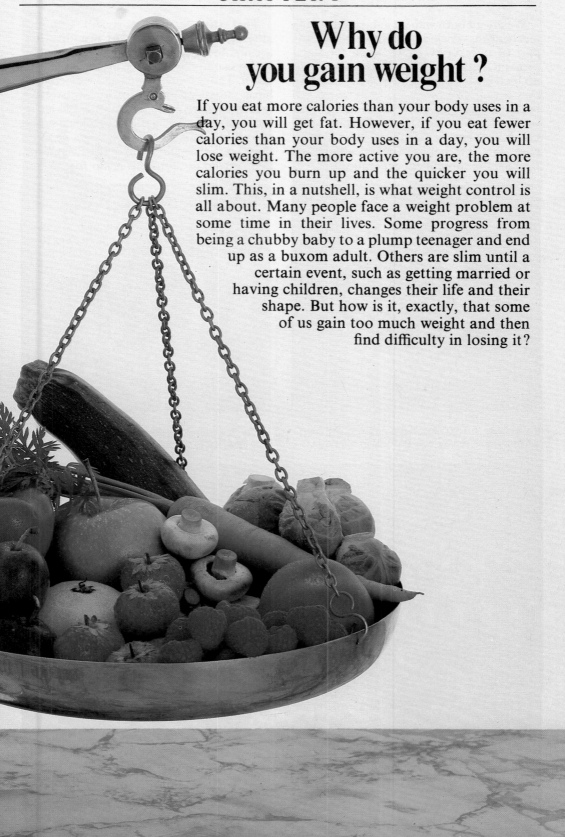

CHAPTER 1

Why do you gain weight?

If you eat more calories than your body uses in a day, you will get fat. However, if you eat fewer calories than your body uses in a day, you will lose weight. The more active you are, the more calories you burn up and the quicker you will slim. This, in a nutshell, is what weight control is all about. Many people face a weight problem at some time in their lives. Some progress from being a chubby baby to a plump teenager and end up as a buxom adult. Others are slim until a certain event, such as getting married or having children, changes their life and their shape. But how is it, exactly, that some of us gain too much weight and then find difficulty in losing it?

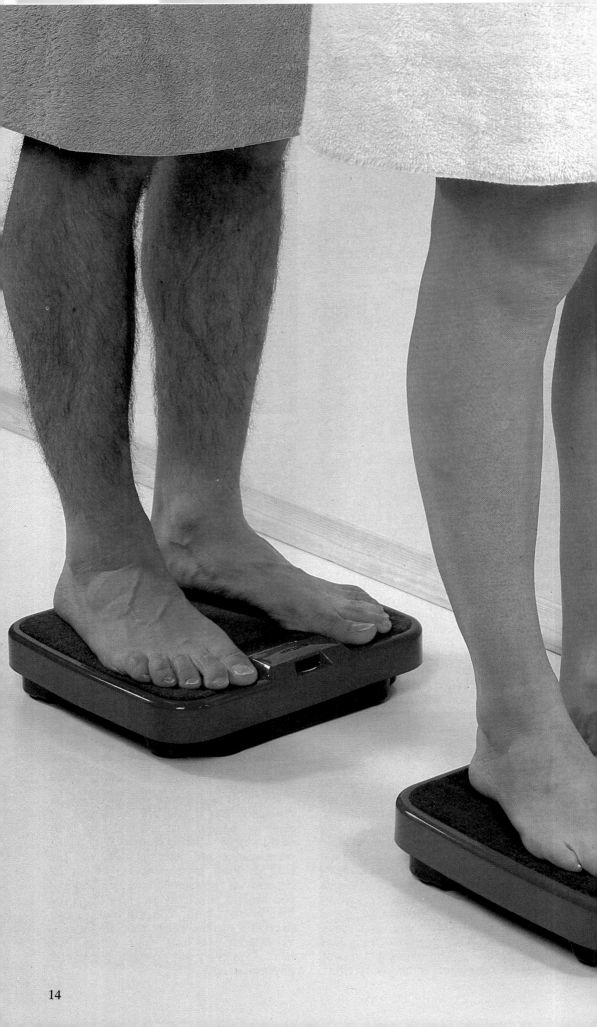

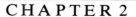
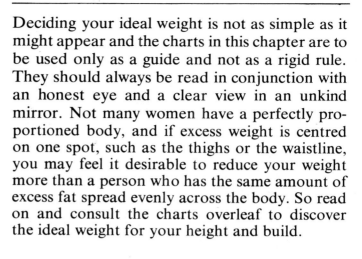

CHAPTER 2

Deciding your ideal weight is not as simple as it might appear and the charts in this chapter are to be used only as a guide and not as a rigid rule. They should always be read in conjunction with an honest eye and a clear view in an unkind mirror. Not many women have a perfectly proportioned body, and if excess weight is centred on one spot, such as the thighs or the waistline, you may feel it desirable to reduce your weight more than a person who has the same amount of excess fat spread evenly across the body. So read on and consult the charts overleaf to discover the ideal weight for your height and build.

What should you weigh?

The right weight for you is governed by your height, and do not take it for granted that you know this accurately. Check it carefully right now instead of relying on an approximate reference from years ago. Professor John Yudkin points out that from about the age of 25 upwards 'you could say it's downhill all the way. Over the years, we are all slowly shrinking. There's a daily height variation, too. You are slightly, but usually measurably, taller first thing in the morning than at the end of the day. Middle-aged slimmers who pinpoint a target weight from the height given on a passport taken out in their twenties could be several pounds adrift; they have probably shrunk into a lower range. Many women who know their weight to the last gram or ounce have never had their height accurately assessed.'

Because there is no such thing as a precise ideal weight, you should use these charts only as a general guide. Your ideal is governed by your skeleton's spread. Neat and narrow body 'scaffolding' will need less cladding than a rangier bone structure. Wrist, hand and foot sizes are not a good guide to frame size, and forget about 'big' bones — it is their *spread* that matters.

Stand in front of a full-length mirror and take a critical look at your figure. You are the best judge of when you are at your ideal weight. If you cannot see any ugly bulges and you can no longer grab any handfuls of fat, then you are at a weight which is right for you. Clothes sizes are not a good indication; manufacturers' sizes differ considerably and your height is also relevant. If you are short, every extra bit of weight seems to show. However, taller women may fluctuate up and down on the scales without anyone but themselves noticing. Compare your weight with the ones given on the following charts. All heights/weights shown are minus shoes, and all weights are to the nearest 0.5kg (1lb). Weights for women and men allow 1.5kg (3lb) for light indoor clothes. Figures for girls and boys are minus clothing. For children under 17, weight is governed by height rather than by age and can be a rough indication only — an immature body grows in spurts and its proportions and shape alter constantly.

If a child appears plump, and a checkout with our chart confirms a call to action, then the emphasis should be on quietly correcting any family and personal eating habits that have caused the damage. Aim not so much at reducing the child's weight but at holding it steady. Then, as his height increases, the child will grow out of the problem.

Weigh with care

It is important to be consistent when weighing yourself. Although there is often a great temptation to leap on the scales every day, try to weigh only once a week on the same scales and at the same time of day. Hourly fluctuations in body weight can mislead you about your slimming progress, and most people are lighter first thing in the morning than in the evening.

Some women may find they weigh 1kg (2-3lb) heavier than they expect (even more, in comparatively rare cases) in the week before their menstrual period. This is due to temporary fluid retention, but such a 'gain' will disappear by the next week's weigh-in. There is no such thing as chronic fluid retention causing surplus weight in a woman who is in otherwise normal health. Plain old 'fat retention' is the problem!

Weigh yourself on good quality scales which are properly adjusted and based on a flat, rigid surface. Readings from scales based on a carpet can be misleading. Stand full-square on your scales because leaning sideways, backwards or forwards can distort the reading. However, if you *must* lean back to make yourself a little 'thinner', remember to do so every time!

Ideal weight charts

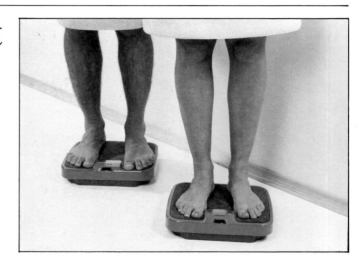

If you are a man

Height is minus shoes and weight includes 1.5kg (3lb) for clothing. Although we give minimum and maximum weights, your ideal will usually be around the average figure or up to 5kg (10lb) more or less, according to your skeletal spread.

Height		Minimum		Ideal average		Maximum	
1.57m	5ft 2in	52.5kg	8st 3lb	57kg	9st 0lb	65.5kg	10st 4lb
1.60m	5ft 3in	53.5kg	8st 6lb	59kg	9st 4lb	66.5kg	10st 7lb
1.63m	5ft 4in	54.5kg	8st 8lb	60.5kg	9st 7lb	68.5kg	10st 11lb
1.65m	5ft 5in	56kg	8st 12lb	61.5kg	9st 10lb	70.5kg	11st 1lb
1.68m	5ft 6in	57.5kg	9st 1lb	63kg	9st 13lb	72kg	11st 4lb
1.70m	5ft 7in	59.5kg	9st 5lb	65kg	10st 3lb	74.5kg	11st 10lb
1.73m	5ft 8in	61kg	9st 8lb	67kg	10st 8lb	77kg	12st 1lb
1.75m	5ft 9in	63kg	9st 13lb	69kg	10st 12lb	78.5kg	12st 5lb
1.78m	5ft 10in	65kg	10st 3lb	71kg	11st 2lb	80.5kg	12st 8lb
1.80m	5ft 11in	66.5kg	10st 7lb	73kg	11st 7lb	82.5kg	13st 0lb
1.83m	6ft 0in	68.5kg	10st 11lb	75kg	11st 11lb	85kg	13st 5lb
1.85m	6ft 1in	70.5kg	11st 1lb	76.5kg	12st 1lb	87kg	13st 10lb
1.88m	6ft 2in	72.5kg	11st 5lb	79kg	12st 6lb	89.5kg	14st 1lb
1.90m	6ft 3in	74kg	11st 6lb	81kg	12st 11lb	92kg	14st 6lb

If you are a woman

Height is minus shoes and weight includes 1.5kg (3lb) for clothing. Although we give minimum and maximum weights, your ideal will usually be around the average figure or up to 5kg (10lb) more or less, according to your skeletal spread.

Height		Minimum		Ideal average		Maximum	
1.47m	4ft 10in	43kg	6st 11lb	47.5kg	7st 7lb	54kg	8st 7lb
1.50m	4ft 11in	44kg	6st 13lb	48.5kg	7st 9lb	56.5kg	8st 13lb
1.52m	5ft 0in	45kg	7st 1lb	50kg	7st 12lb	58kg	9st 2lb
1.55m	5ft 1in	46.5kg	7st 4lb	51.5kg	8st 1lb	59.5kg	9st 5lb
1.57m	5ft 2in	47.5kg	7st 7lb	52.5kg	8st 4lb	61kg	9st 8lb
1.60m	5ft 3in	49kg	7st 10lb	54kg	8st 7lb	62kg	9st 11lb
1.63m	5ft 4in	50.5kg	7st 13lb	56kg	8st 11lb	64kg	10st 1lb
1.65m	5ft 5in	51.5kg	8st 2lb	57kg	9st 0lb	66kg	10st 5lb
1.68m	5ft 6in	53kg	8st 5lb	59.5kg	9st 5lb	67.5kg	10st 9lb
1.70m	5ft 7in	55kg	8st 9lb	61kg	9st 9lb	69.5kg	10st 13lb
1.73m	5ft 8in	56.5kg	8st 13lb	63kg	9st 13lb	71.5kg	11st 3lb
1.75m	5ft 9in	58.5kg	9st 3lb	65kg	10st 3lb	73kg	11st 7lb
1.78m	5ft 10lb	60.5kg	9st 7lb	66.5kg	10st 7lb	75.5kg	11st 12lb
1.80m	5ft 11in	62kg	9st 11lb	68.5kg	10st 11lb	77.5kg	12st 3lb
1.83m	6ft 0in	64kg	10st 1lb	70.5kg	11st 1lb	80kg	12st 8lb

If you are a boy under 17

Height		Lowest		Highest		Approx. age
1.10m	3ft 7in	17kg	2st 10lb	22kg	3st 7lb	5
1.15m	3ft 9in	18kg	2st 12lb	25kg	3st 13lb	6
1.22m	4ft 0in	21kg	3st 4lb	28.5kg	4st 7lb	7
1.29m	4ft 3in	22.5kg	3st 8lb	33kg	5st 3lb	8
1.35m	4ft 5in	26kg	4st 1lb	36.5kg	5st 10lb	9
1.39m	4ft 7in	27.5kg	4st 5lb	40kg	6st 4lb	10
1.45m	4ft 9in	28.5kg	4st 7lb	43.5kg	6st 12lb	11
1.47m	4ft 10in	32kg	5st 1lb	48kg	7st 8lb	12
1.53m	5ft 0in	34kg	5st 5lb	54kg	8st 7lb	13
1.60m	5ft 3in	39kg	6st 2lb	61kg	9st 9lb	14
1.65m	5ft 5in	44.5kg	7st 0lb	62kg	9st 11lb	15
1.68m	5ft 6in	49.5kg	7st 11lb	67kg	10st 8lb	16

If you are a girl under 17

Height		Lowest		Highest		Approx. age
1.10m	3ft 7in	17kg	2st 10lb	21.5kg	3st 5lb	5
1.15m	3ft 9in	18.5kg	2st 13lb	23.5kg	3st 10lb	6
1.19m	3ft 11in	20.5kg	3st 3lb	24.5kg	3st 12lb	7
1.24m	4ft 1in	22.5kg	3st 8lb	30.5kg	4st 11lb	8
1.27m	4ft 2in	23.5kg	3st 10lb	34.5kg	5st 6lb	9
1.35m	4ft 5in	26.5kg	4st 2lb	40kg	6st 4lb	10
1.42m	4ft 8in	28kg	4st 6lb	45kg	7st 1lb	11
1.47m	4ft 10in	30kg	4st 10lb	49.5kg	7st 11lb	12
1.55m	5ft 1in	36.5kg	5st 11lb	54kg	8st 7lb	13
1.57m	5ft 2in	41.3kg	6st 7lb	55.5kg	8st 10lb	14
1.60m	5ft 3in	45.5kg	7st 2lb	57kg	9st 0lb	15
1.63m	5ft 4in	46.5kg	7st 4lb	58.5kg	9st 3lb	16

WEIGHT MASTERCHARTS

One method used by scientists for measuring excess fat is the calliper test. The flesh is pinched between callipers on four areas of the body: the arms, back, thighs and waist. These measurements are then calculated to give a good idea of how much weight could be dieted away. We measured the twelve women pictured here and show the results the calliper test revealed. Taller women always carry excess weight a lot easier than smaller women, but they may have a bigger frame which cannot be altered by dieting. Most women tend to have particular problem areas, such as the stomach or bottom, and unfortunately there is no guarantee that these problems will disappear completely when they reach their target weight. However, exercise can help to firm and tone saggy muscles.

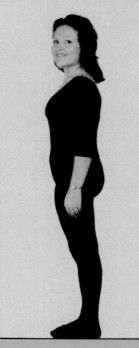

Joyce
1.52m (5ft 0in)
Weighs 51.7kg (8st 2lb)
Surplus 3.2kg (7lb)

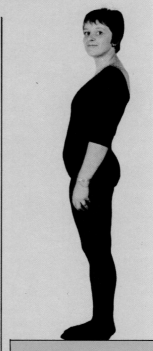

Christine
1.57m (5ft 2in)
Weighs 60.8kg (9st 8lb)
Surplus 5kg (11lb)

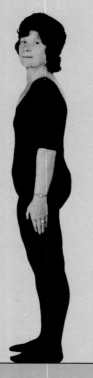

Hilda
1.68m (5ft 6in)
Weighs 70.5kg (11st 1½lb)
Surplus 6.3kg (1st)

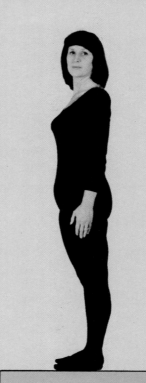

Sheila
1.68m (5ft 6in)
Weighs 62.4kg (9st 11½lb)
Surplus 1.8kg (4lb)

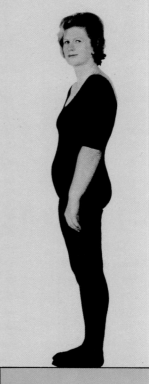

Mary
1.73m (5ft 8in)
Weighs 69.9kg (11st)
Surplus 9.5kg (1st 7lb)

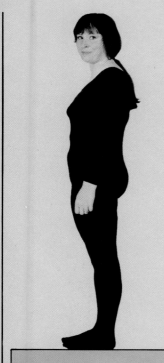

Denise
1.57m (5ft 2in)
Weighs 69.4kg (10st 13lb)
Surplus 12.7kg (2st)

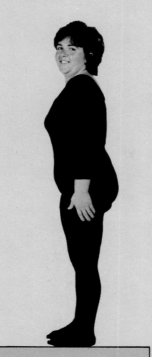

Rosemary
1.60m (5ft 3in)
Weighs 79.8kg (12st 8lb)
Surplus 19.1kg (3st)

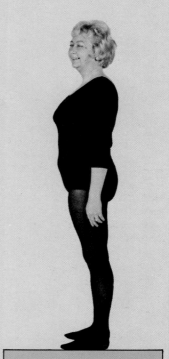

Anne
1.63m (5ft 4in)
Weighs 67.8kg (10st 9½lb)
Surplus 8.6kg (1st 5lb)

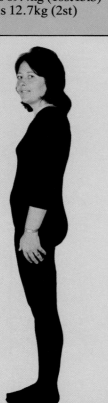

Stephanie
1.73m (5ft 8in)
Weighs 72.2kg (11st 5lb)
Surplus 2.3kg (5lb)

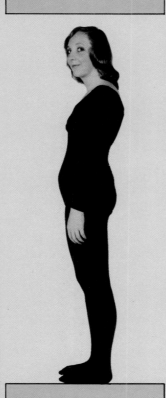

Margaret
1.75m (5ft 9in)
Weighs 73.2kg (11st 7½lb)
Surplus 6.3kg (1st)

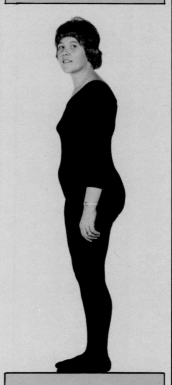

Stella
1.75m (5ft 9in)
Weighs 77.8kg (12st 3½lb)
Surplus 9.5kg (1st 7lb)

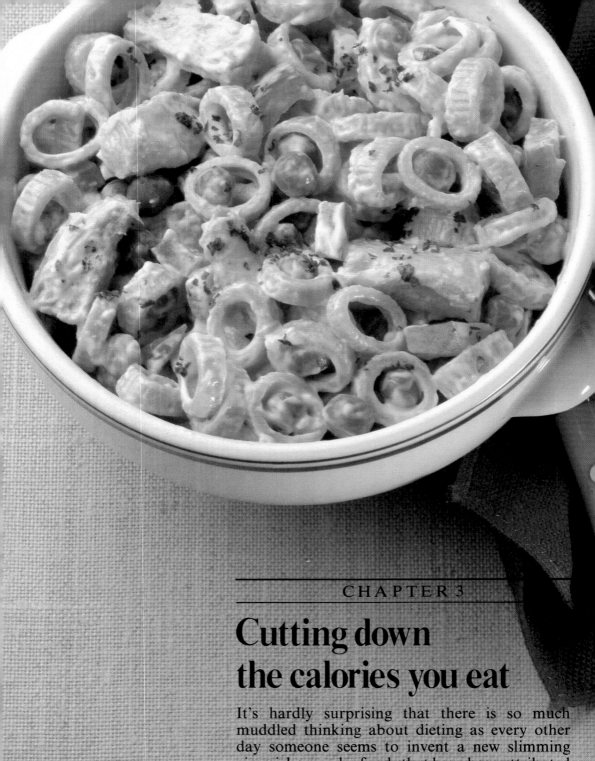

CHAPTER 3

Cutting down the calories you eat

It's hardly surprising that there is so much muddled thinking about dieting as every other day someone seems to invent a new slimming gimmick: wonder foods that have been attributed with magical qualities they in no way deserve; crash diets that guarantee a huge surplus weight loss in a matter of days. Because losing surplus weight is never easy, even seasoned slimmers may be willing to give gimmicks a try just in case there is a magic answer to their weight problem.

Although crash diets may work in the short term, they fail to have any lasting effect on a weight problem. They are usually too rigid to maintain over a long period, and it is not recommended that anyone should diet for longer than a couple of weeks on an allowance of less than

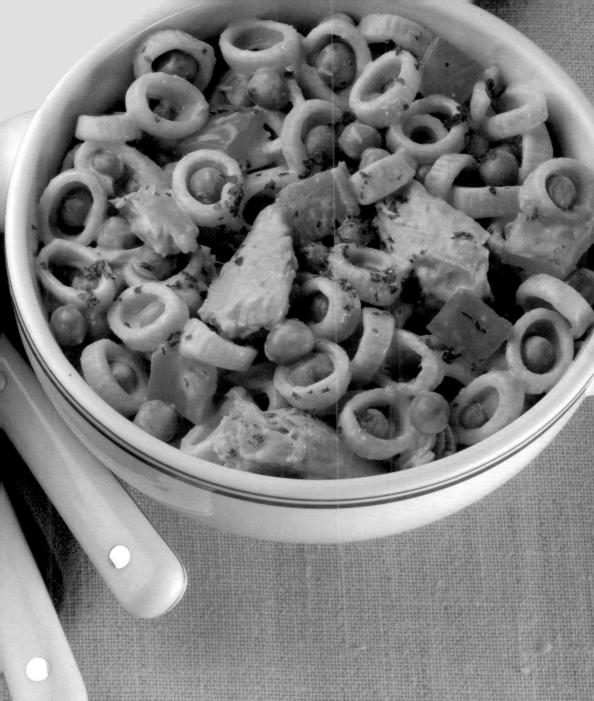

1,000 calories a day. If you do not supply your body with all the nutrients it needs, you will probably become less active and more tired than normal. This, in turn, means that you will start using up fewer calories a day and so the crash diet eventually becomes counter-productive. All the foods that you eat, and most drinks, contain calories, and no food or drink can create a special chemical reaction in the body which will 'melt' away the unwanted fat.

The unassailable truth is that, no matter what you eat, the key to losing weight is to limit the number of calories you take in. Whether you choose to do this by counting calories, or by following a high-fibre diet or a low-fat diet, the result will be the same.

Although these two dishes may look the same, the salad on the left contains 415 more calories than the special low-calorie version on the right. In order to achieve this, we used low-calorie salad dressing instead of mayonnaise, and tuna in brine instead of tuna in oil. So cutting down on calories does not mean that you have to eat less. Turn to page 136 for the recipe for the low-calorie version of this delicious dish — Wholewheat Pasta and Tuna Salad.

Calorie-controlled diets

Counting every calorie is the surest way to lose weight but it demands precision: all foods must be weighed and calculated and their calories then added together to make up your daily allowance. Guess-work *won't* work. A pair of kitchen scales that weighs small amounts accurately is an essential piece of slimming equipment. You also need a jug that will measure liquids in fluid ounces or down to 25ml. Accurate measuring spoons, in either metric or imperial measurements, should be used rather than the nearest spoon that comes to hand in your cutlery drawer. Just 7g ($\frac{1}{4}$oz) butter comes to 52 calories, 5ml (1 teaspoon) oil is 40 calories, and 28g (1oz) Cheddar cheese is 120 calories, so guessing by eye could mean a big calorie miscalculation. A few wrong guesses during the day and you may prevent yourself losing any weight at all. It is also worth writing down everything you eat. It is surprisingly easy to develop a form of amnesia about foods and, in particular, drinks which you have consumed. Calorie counters tend to organize their dieting in one of two ways: some plan out their day's eating in advance, calculate their calories before they start, and keep to just those foods; others allot themselves a calorie total and deduct the calories as they eat them. The danger with the latter method, of course, is that you have to beware of being too generous with your calories early in the day in order to leave yourself an adequate calorie allowance for the evening meal.

The great advantage of counting calories is that you can eat absolutely anything you fancy as long as it does not exceed your allowance. Although a set diet may try to cater for differing lifestyles and tastes, it is likely that there will be at least one food you dislike, or one which is difficult to purchase. However, if you know your calories, you can substitute a food of equal calories.

If you do not wish to follow a set diet you can easily construct your own using the calorie charts at the end of this book. The best diet for you is the one you find easiest to follow and that which fits most neatly into your own lifestyle. But remember to take care to make your diet as varied as possible and to include lots of foods which have a high nutritional value.

It is worth trying to learn the approximate calorific values of your favourite basic foods by heart; once they are memorized you will find it easier to make a diet-wise choice in restaurants or when you are away from home. You will learn which foods you must avoid and which foods are filling and satisfying for little calorie cost. Absorbing these few initial facts will not only help you to lose weight now but will also make it easier for you to stay slim.

The diets in this book count the calories for you in various ways. Designed to fit a variety of lifestyles and patterns of eating, these diets cater for all tastes and figures. The diet-package plan does all the thinking for you. Each diet is worked out in detail from the first bite to the last crumb and is balanced carefully to give you a good supply of all the essential nutrients. As a general rule, if you are over 18kg (3st) overweight (see the charts in *What should you weigh?*), start off on a 1,500 calorie a day diet. However, if you have less than 6kg (1st) to lose, you will need to keep to 1,000 calories. Whether you choose 1,000, 1,250 or 1,500 calories a day, provided you eat precisely what you are told and weigh out all foods accurately, then weight loss should follow.

The low-fat diet

Fats *are* fattening – they're the highest-calorie foods of all – and that is why low-fat dieting has become a very successful method of losing weight. By reducing your fats intake you are indirectly controlling your calories, and you will slim in a healthy way.

Low-fat dieting has been greeted with unqualified support in both medical and nutritional worlds. The Royal College of Physicians, the British Cardiac Society and top nutritional experts in the United States have all recommended an overall reduction of fat in British and American diets.

In recent years, nutritionists have found a direct parallel between the percentage of fats in national diets and the prevalence of weight problems. In countries where the diet contains a very high percentage of fat (America, for instance), obesity has become a health problem of epidemic proportions. In countries where the diet is marginally less fatty (as in some northern European countries, for instance), the obesity problem is correspondingly less severe. But in those countries where the basic diet is very low in fat (Korea, for instance, where fat accounts for only 8 per cent of daily calorie intake), obesity is extremely rare.

The most widely-agreed picture of an ideal healthy diet is one that is low in fats, particularly the animal fats. Doctors looking into the causes of heart disease have found now that an important factor may be the concentration of fat-like substances in the blood stream. This is affected by what we eat and it is thought that reducing fat in our food can help to prevent the build-up of fatty deposits in the blood. A healthy diet should contain a generous quantity of high-fibre foods. It should be low in sugar, which has little to offer other than calories and is a factor in dental decay. It should provide a generous quantity of fruit and vegetables. When you follow the new low-fat method of dieting you will automatically follow the same pattern as that recommended for good health.

The low-fat diet is very successful as a reducing diet because, by controlling the intake of fats, it also controls automatically your intake of the highest-calorie foods. If you look at the calorie chart, you will see, that such fats as butter and lard are much higher in calories than carbohydrate foods. You will notice also that fatty meats and cheeses contain more calories than do low-fat meats and cheeses, and the lowest-calorie foods of all are those that contain no fat.

An astonishing number of innocent-looking foods contain 'invisible' fats; and although it is easy to see and remove the fat from the outside of a slice of ham or a lamb chop, it is more difficult to identify fat if it is hidden in biscuits, cakes or cheese. In order to slim effectively using this method, you must be aware of the invisible fat in foods. The pioneer low-fat method, as devised by *Slimming Magazine*, allocates a fat unit number to each food according to the amount of fat it contains. Hundreds of basic foods have been analyzed to provide this information. On this diet, you are allowed up to 10 fat units a day and have access to a wide range of 'free foods'.

This diet's popularity lies in its utter simplicity. There is no need to count every single calorie — as long as you keep to your allowance of 10 fat units each day it is unlikely that you could eat enough free food calories to prevent your losing any weight. Switches from high-fat foods to lower-fat foods are often effortless and non-sacrificial. By changing from 75g (3oz) Cheddar cheese (10½ fat units) with your salad to 75g (3oz) roast skinless chicken (1½ fat units) you will save 235 calories. If you switched to 75g (3oz) prawns (¼ fat unit) instead, you would save another 35 calories. Fruits and vegetables are unrationed, and cereals, rice and pasta are allowed in generous quantities, so that you will always get the filling, healthy fibre you need.

Many slimmers are delighted by the results they have had by following this diet. Not only have they become slim but they are also staying slim, because they continue to follow some of the fat-cutting habits they learned on the diet.

The high-fibre diet

Eat more dietary fibre. That's the message coming loud and clear from leading medical and nutritional experts in the Western world. And since *Slimming Magazine's* own Audrey Eyton first published her famous *F-Plan Diet* in the early 1980s, there can be few people who have *not* heard about dietary fibre and its slimming and health benefits.

It has been shown that a diet rich in dietary fibre offers real advantages for both health and weight control. But what is dietary fibre and what is meant by a high-fibre diet? Essentially, dietary fibre is the carbohydrate material found in plant foods, mainly in the cell walls, which is not digested by man. It used to be called 'roughage' and is found in everyday plant foods to a greater or lesser extent. For example, wholemeal bread, bran cereals, potatoes, peas, beans, sweetcorn, spinach, raspberries, figs and many other fruits and vegetables contain appreciable amounts of dietary fibre.

High-fibre foods also happen to be the kind that will fill you up, and are therefore extremely satisfying for a slimmer to eat. It doesn't take long for a fibre-free glass of fruit juice or piece of cheese to slip down, but you can't say that about a juicy orange or a bowl of crunchy bran flakes!

Another benefit of a high-fibre diet is that high-fibre foods tend to need more chewing and swallowing than low-fibre ones because they are bulky and have plenty of texture. This means a high-fibre diet can slow down your eating considerably. And, because dietary fibre is not completely digested, some calories in the food are excreted with the fibre.

High-fibre meals tend to be nicely-filling because dietary fibre soaks up water and makes the food swell to a large volume in the stomach. With a full stomach, you will not feel hungry and there will be less temptation to eat more than you are allowed. In addition, high-fibre foods do not cause 'rebound hunger'. This particularly occurs after meals consisting of refined carbohydrates, when the food eaten causes the blood sugar level to rise very quickly. The body then produces insulin, which drops it down to pre-meal levels, leaving you feeling hungrier than you were before. This rebound hypoglycaemic effect does not occur with natural, fibre-rich foods, which are converted more slowly into blood sugar.

In order to lose weight, you will probably need to control your intake of calories as well as increase your intake of fibre. But by increasing your daily intake of dietary fibre to between 35g and 50g a day and by following a calorie-counted or low-fat diet plan, you should be able to slim extra-easily and effectively.

As well as the slimming effects of a high-fibre diet, there are appreciable health advantages, too. There is convincing evidence that a diet rich in dietary fibre can reduce the risk of some of the major diseases of the Western world, such as coronary heart disease, cancer of the large bowel, diabetes, diverticulitis and other bowel disorders such as constipation and haemorrhoids. Medical and scientific research in developing countries has firmly established a link between dietary habits and disease patterns. People in those countries eat a very high-fibre diet and are virtually unafflicted by the Western degenerative diseases. Western societies, on

Is it necessary to weigh everything when you count calories?
The really low-calorie vegetables are the only safe exceptions. Here you see a small plate of salad vegetables (no oily dressing, of course) and a large plate. We also picture a modest serving of Brussels sprouts and a more generous one. In each case, the calories added by extra generosity are not significant enough to make any difference to daily weight loss.

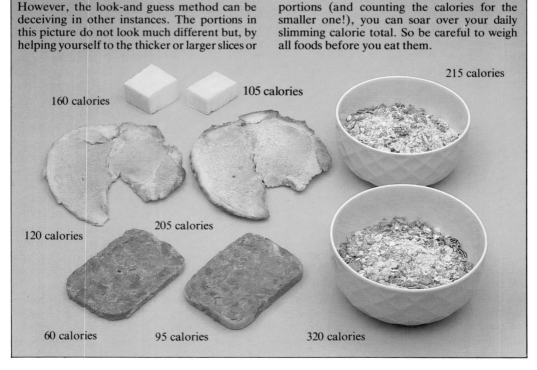

35 calories

20 calories

20 calories

45 calories

However, the look-and guess method can be deceiving in other instances. The portions in this picture do not look much different but, by helping yourself to the thicker or larger slices or portions (and counting the calories for the smaller one!), you can soar over your daily slimming calorie total. So be careful to weigh all foods before you eat them.

215 calories

160 calories

105 calories

120 calories

205 calories

60 calories

95 calories

320 calories

Is dry sherry less fattening than sweet sherry?

In this picture are equal calorie quantities of sweet and dry sherry (55 calories), and sweet and dry wine (75 calories), As you see, you do get a little more for your calories by choosing the 'dry' drinks — but it's only a small saving. However, it is better to drink dry versions whenever possible both to reduce calories and curb your 'sweet tooth'.

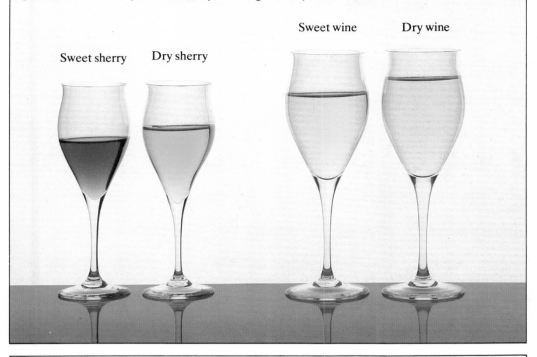

Sweet sherry   Dry sherry   Sweet wine   Dry wine

Is wine less fattening than spirits ?

Yes, if you drink the same quantity of wine as spirits. On the left, in the picture, is a bar single measure of whisky (50 calories) and the same quantity of dry white wine (only 16 calories). On the right, you can see the calories in a small 113ml (4floz) glass, and a medium 142ml (5floz) measure and a large 170ml (6 floz) measure of wine. All have more calories than a glass of spirits when you take into account the vital factors of 'normal quantity' — unless you are in the habit of pouring doubles.

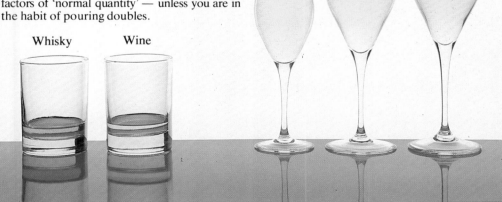

Whisky   Wine   75 calories   95 calories   110 calories

the other hand, eat far more fat, mostly of animal origin, and very little dietary fibre. In addition, obesity is uncommon in developing countries, but is extremely prevalent in countries like Britain, Australia and the United States.

You can use the charts at the back of this book to compile your own high-fibre diet — or follow one of our diet plans making sure you select the meals which are highest in fibre. The minimum amount of fibre you should be aiming for each day is 35 g and in order to lose weight you will also need to keep calories between 1,000 and 1,500 a day (see page 12) or, if you are following a low-fat diet, keep fat units to 10 a day.

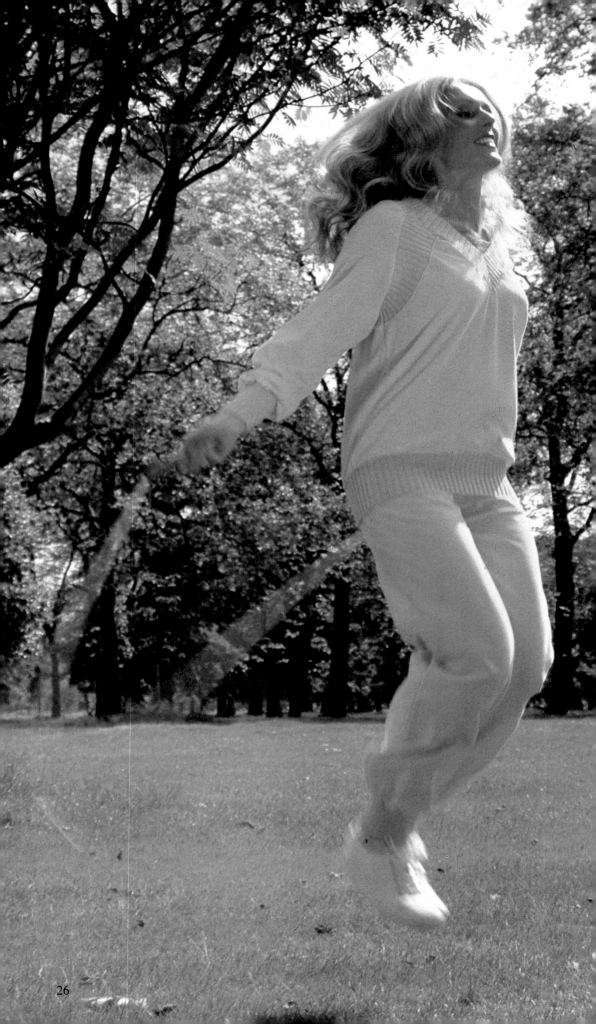

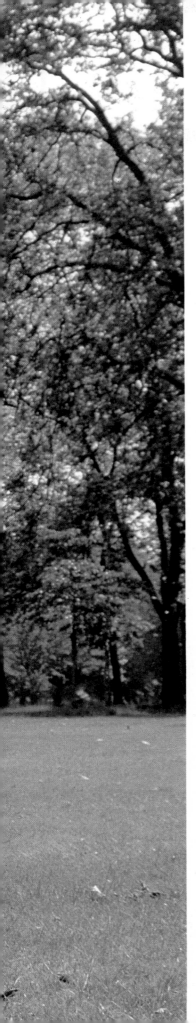

CHAPTER 4

Increasing the amount of exercise you take can be an effective booster for your dieting campaign. When you are slimming, your basic aim is to eat fewer calories than your body needs each day so that it has to draw on its fatty reserves for energy. You can do this by diet alone: restricting the calories your body takes in. However, if by extra physical activity you also boost your body's daily calorie-output rate, you are attacking your weight problem on two fronts, by diet and exercise.

Stepping up the calories you burn

Building a regular exercise routine into your life could bene-fit your health as well as help you into shape. Exercise has many other positive benefits, too, such as making you feel good. So it's worth making the effort even if you have always considered yourself unsporty. Although we have little control over our basal metabolic rate — the number of calories our body needs simply to maintain all its functions — we do control the number of calories we expend on activities. And, even if you don't take up sport or do particular exercises, it is possible to increase your calorie burn-up significantly by tackling tasks more energetically and by seizing every chance to walk, climb stairs and generally move extra-briskly. Yes, some people do have high basal meta-bolic rates, while others have lower rates. But it is in the number of calories used up in activities throughout the day that scientists have observed the most striking differences.

Some people seem to be born with greater exercise resist-ance than others. Scientists have discovered that variations are apparent even in young babies. Whereas there are lazy babies who lie peacefully in their cots, there are also active babies who wriggle and roll about. These differences in activity levels tend to continue throughout childhood and even into adulthood. Even when it comes to ordinary house-hold tasks, exercise-resistant people will find ways to minimize movement and they may be quite unaware of their bodies' artful ploys to save calories.

Physical activity is a term that embraces all bodily move-ment. It not only includes what we normally think of as being 'exercise', such as running, sports and keep-fit exercises, but it also takes in shopping, climbing the stairs and even walking across the room. In fact, every time we move we are burning up at least some calories. These days, weight control experts advocate that you should weave more total body movement into your everyday activity rather than concentrating on setting aside a period of time for special exercises. The former, they advise, is what really helps when you are aiming at lasting weight control. It is the sum total of the little movements during the course of the day that has the most significant effect on calorie expenditure and, therefore, on weight. You can observe the truth of this yourself — almost certainly among your acquaintances there will be a woman who is described as being 'full of nervous energy'. She is almost invariably lean. Watch her closely next time you visit her home. See how many times she rises from her seat to perform some task or to fetch something. Observe how brisk all her movements tend to be. It is likely, too, that your friends include at least one heavily overweight woman who swears that she does not eat a lot and cannot understand why she weighs so much — she is best observed doing housework. Although she might be coping with a busy day, see how little she actually moves in performing her household tasks, and how slowly she moves. Without being aware of it, she has devised methods of performing each task that involve a minimum of body movement. When she settles into her armchair, note her tendency to call on other people to fetch something she needs from the next room, rather than get up and fetch it herself.

Even apparently young and fit people who take up some form of sport can still be exercise resistant. Some ball games, for example, offer great opportunities for being idle and standing around when you may be tricked into thinking you have exercised hard and steadily. Watch some people on a tennis court — while some players rush around the court burning up calories, others move slowly and practise only right-arm activity!

Unfortunately the whole concept of exercise breeds great resistance in many women, particularly those with a weight problem. Anyone who has been a plump child still remembers the horror of games and the humiliations of the

You can step up your general level of activity and exercise anywhere without recourse to special equipment, clothing or surroundings. Just wear some casual, loose-fitting clothing (track suits, shorts and leotards are ideal) and practise some bending and stretching exercises to loosen up and relax stiff, aching limbs and tone up sagging muscles. Details of special exercises for shaping up thighs, stomach, bottom and arms are given in Chapter 9: Getting into shape. If you prefer not to exercise alone, then seek the moral support and guidance of others and join a local gym or keep-fit and dancing classes.

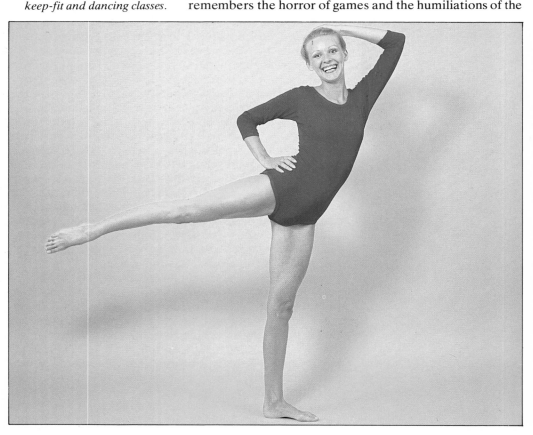

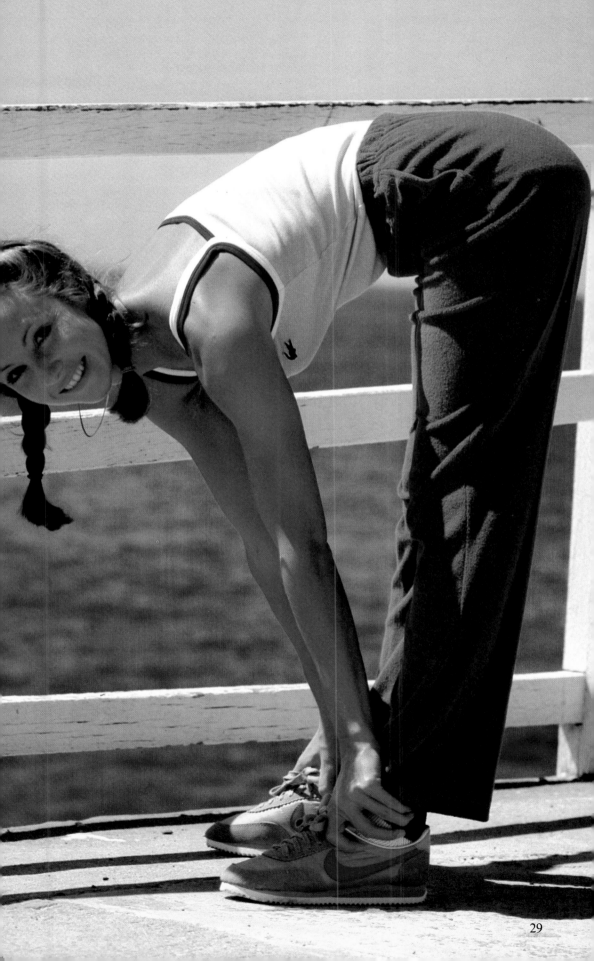

school gym. Furthermore, most of us have an in-built guilt complex about exercise which we know we ought to do, always intend to do, but never quite get round to doing. In the following pages, we outline a plan of campaign for all exercise haters.

Beating activity resistance

You can start tackling the task of increasing your daily calorie output in the simplest of ways. Begin, perhaps, by concentrating on speeding up both your movements and activities. Break your age-old habits and walk more swiftly — it will soon become habitual to you, whether you are popping out to the shops, walking to a neighbour's home or just ambling around the house.

You can also work at changing your attitude towards physical activity and exertion. Instead of cursing the fact that you must climb upstairs to fetch something, start to welcome that extra climb as an opportunity to burn a few more calories. Also, try to speed up your rate of ascent each time you go upstairs. Begin to embrace every natural opportunity to move, however small it is. This, too, will gradually become quite effortless. The 'nervous energy' person is quite unaware of the movement in her day — to her, it is effortless and natural. You, too, with a little initial effort, can become more active and less conscious of the movements you perform.

Every time we move, we are burning up at least some calories. The more parts of our bodies that we move, the more calories we burn up. Hence, moving your whole body from place to place by walking will burn up considerably more calories than simply moving one arm to iron or two hands to type. The speed at which we move also affects the number of calories we burn. The faster the movement, the greater the number of calories used. Thus brisk walking burns significantly more calories than strolling, and jogging or running burn more than a brisk walk. The third factor that affects the number of calories burned by body movement is the pull of gravity; walking upstairs or uphill will use up more calories than proceeding along level

Badminton (below) and squash (right) are good sports for burning up calories. Although badminton is a gentler game than the faster, hard-hitting squash racquets, it still involves a lot of movement on the court and stretching and reaching for the shuttlecock as it darts backwards and forwards across the net. Most sports clubs and local community centres cater for both these sports although you can, of course, rig up a badminton net in your own back garden and practise with your family and friends.

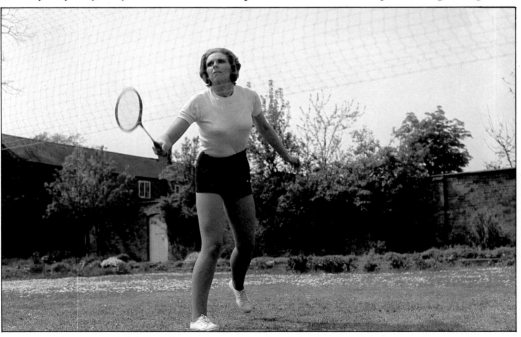

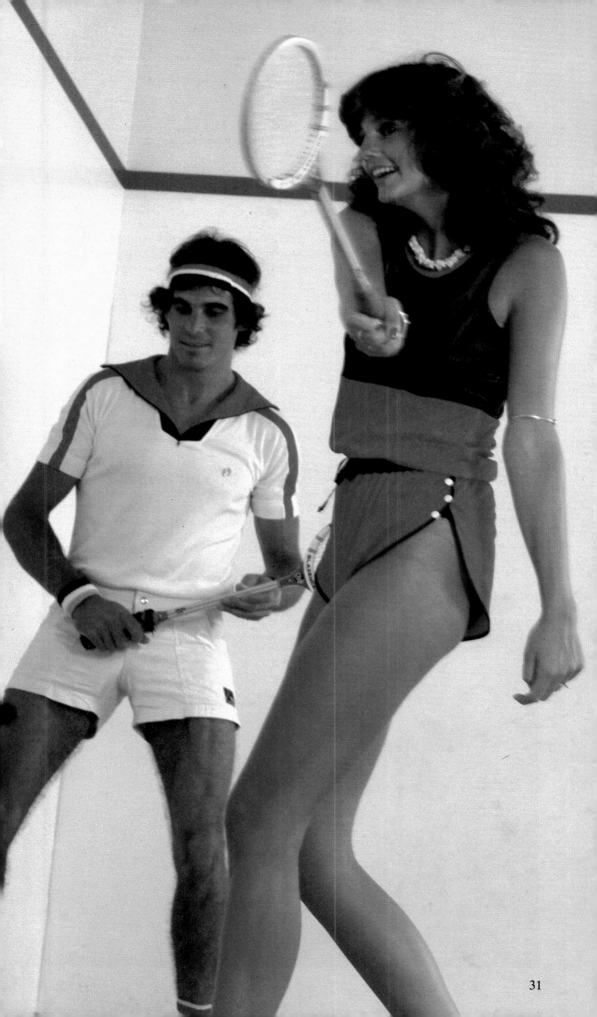

ground. So the activities that produce the maximum in calorie burn-up are those that involve moving the whole body, at a fast pace, in an upwards direction, such as running uphill, rushing upstairs or skipping. Climbing stairs more than usual will incorporate a great deal of high-calorie-burning activity into your routine. Resist the temptation to ask other people to fetch and carry for you, and get up and go yourself at the briskest possible pace. Before you embark on any task, consider how you can do it with the maximum amount of body movement. One bonus of being overweight is that you burn up more calories taking exercise than a slim person. This is because more calories are needed to move a heavier body.

Once you have made a start on increasing your energy output, you will soon notice the positive results. Add to it, as you go along, by introducing some deliberate exercise into your usual daily routine. Instead of driving or bussing to a regular destination like the shops or the station, walk briskly. These additional walks will supplement the increase of movement in your small daily activities and thus boost the overall calorie expenditure.

If an overweight person takes a brisk walk for 30 minutes each day for a year, it could add up to a considerable weight loss — even up to 6kg(1st) a year, in addition to the amount you lose by dieting. You could also lose that extra weight if you cycled for 20 minutes to the shops or work and then back again, five days a week. Both walking and cycling can also play a useful role in the prevention of coronary attacks. It does not matter that only your legs are being exercised — in terms of coronary circulation, exercising any part of your body affects the whole circulation of your blood. However, if you are very overweight, you should refrain from pedalling hard up enormous hills — any violent exercise is unwise for an unfit person.

Having started to think in terms of calorie output, it may be a good idea to take up some form of sporting activity that appeals to you or which you used to enjoy in the past. Remember that in order to be enjoyed, sports do not have

Walking is the simplest and easiest activity of all and a great way of burning up excess calories. Make walking an integral part of your daily routine either by going out for a special walk or by walking when you would normally drive or catch a bus. At weekends, plan a long walk in the countryside or a local park — you will find it relaxing and enjoyable.

In addition to boosting your slimming campaign, walking is a good method of alleviating boredom — an escape route from the house when you might otherwise be tempted to eat illicit, fattening snack meals.

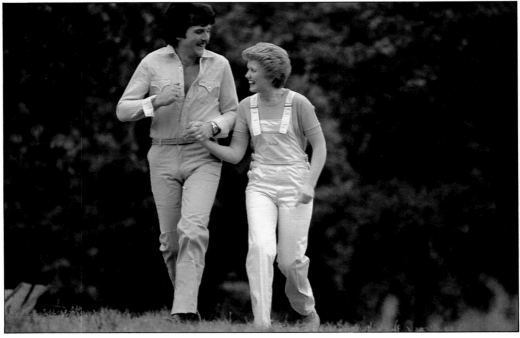

The A to Z of calorie expenditure

Even when you are sleeping or sitting down and doing nothing, your body is burning calories to keep your lungs breathing, your heart beating, your blood circulating and your body functioning generally. However, this is only the minimum number of calories you can burn. Once you start moving your body in any way, you burn more calories. The following chart shows how many calories you use up in different forms of activity.

The rate at which we burn calories while we are physically at rest is called the 'basal metabolic rate'. Scientific research has now shown that the average woman burns up calories at a rate of about one calorie per minute just on body maintenance, even when resting or lying in bed. Remember, though, that this figure is an average and some people have a lower metabolic rate, burning less than one calorie per minute, while others will have a higher than average metabolic rate.

However, when it comes to the extra calories burned up in physical activity, overweight people have an advantage. In walking, or in any exercise that involves moving the whole body from place to place,

they burn up more calories per minute than do slim people. The reason is very simple: the heavier a body, the more energy (in the form of calories) that is needed to move it.

The calorie figures in the chart are based on the average expenditure by a woman of average weight. An average man will use up a half calorie a minute more on light exercise to one calorie more on strenuous sports. You can expect to burn up a little more in the way of calories if you are carrying extra fat, but never over-estimate! Even average normal-weight people show differences in the way they tackle various tasks and exercises; some put far more energy into them than others do. It is fairly safe to say that, no matter what weight you are, if you go about your daily activities in an unhurried way your calorie expenditure will be about average as shown in these charts. If you do things slowly and rest rather a lot between activities, it may well be lower. Alternatively if you tackle everything very energetically, moving quickly about your daily tasks, it will be higher. The figures given for a wide range of activities in the accompanying chart are for calories burned up per minute.

Calories used per minute

Archery
A pleasant pastime, but it is mostly arms-only activity plus leisurely walking   3

Athletics
Can be extremely strenuous for short periods of time. During training count   7

Badminton
Playing with average effort, you would run about a lot   5

Basketball
Lots of very fast running, jumping and stretching   7

Bedmaking
Real bends and stretches with sheets and blankets   3

Bends and stretches
On-the-spot exercises such as touching your toes, knee-bends, and so on   3

Billiards
A game that is mostly arm movement. Alas, concentration does not burn calories   2

Bowls
A leisurely sport with little speed, but some bending   3

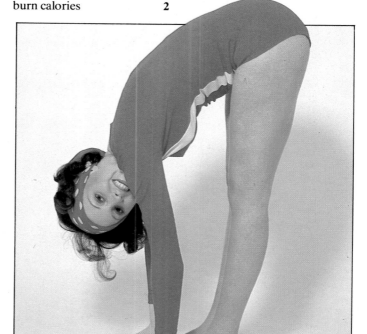

ACTIVITY

Canoeing
Paddling down the river at
3km (2 miles) an hour   3
Racing along at about 6km
(4 miles) an hour   6

Card games
Sitting and puzzling uses
few calories and you only
add the occasional flick
of the wrists   *under* 2

Circuit training
Climbing gymnasium bars,
jumping over the vaulting-
horse and other equipment,
all very strenuous
exercise   10

Cleaning
Cupboards and drawers,
mostly arm movement *under* 2
Floors, with mop or broom
and some walking   3
Windows, if lots of bending
and stretching is involved   3

Climbing
Rock climbing and hill walking
are very strenuous and
enthusiasts keep going for
many hours. Walking up
sloping terrain   6
Tackling arduous rock
faces   *up to* 12

Cooking
Does not involve much
strenuous physical effort
and consists mostly of arm
movements   2

Cricket
If you are fielding   *under* 2
If you are batting or
bowling, the calorie output
should rise   4

Croquet
Another leisurely game that
does not demand strenuous
activity   3

Cross-country running
Marathon events can last for
three or four hours so lots of
calories are consumed   7

Cycling
At a pleasant easy pace
along the straight   5
Strenuously, enthusiastic
style   10

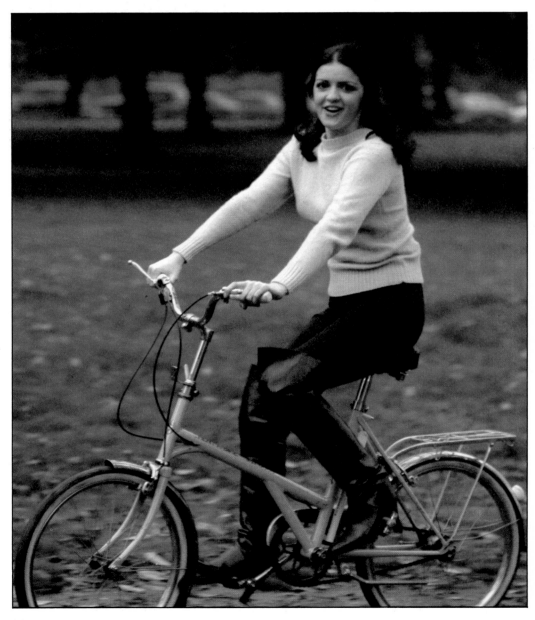

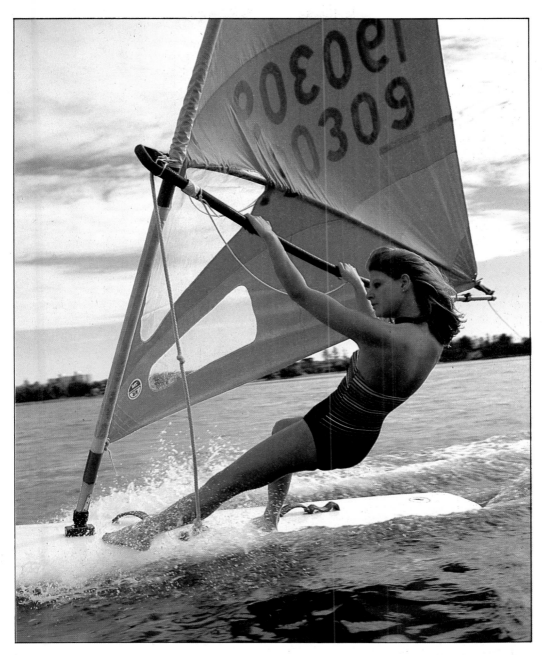

steady but enough to make you want to stop for a breather sometimes **6+**

Washing
Dishes *under* **2**
Clothes by hand. The heavier they are, the more calories you burn **3**

Windsurfing
The more you fall off, the higher your calorie expenditure *up to* **6**

Yoga
With average bending and stretching **3**

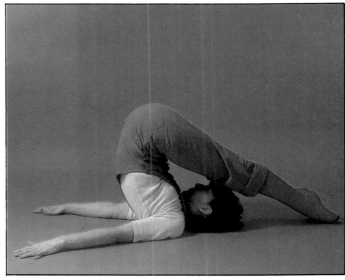

Skip away the weight

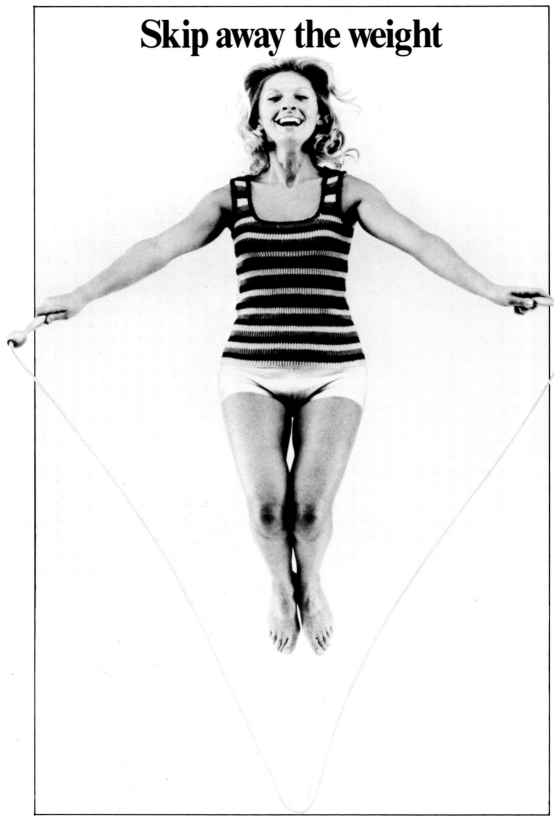

Skipping will use up around 10 calories a minute, and the heavier you are the more calories you burn. It is best to start slowly and just do about 50 skips forwards on your first day (do 25 if that is all you can manage), then add 50 skips a day until you feel able to try some of these skipping exercises.

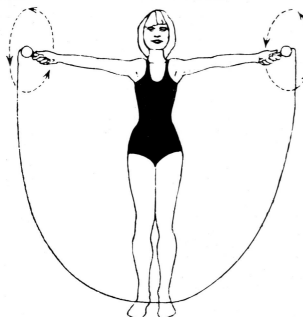

Simple backwards skip ▲

Get your skipping rope, circle handles round backwards, jump up and down with your feet together and skip. Have a long enough skipping rope so that you do not have to drop your arms to jump over it. The higher you keep your arms all the time, the better for muscle firming. It is highly unlikely that you will be able to carry on for half an hour non-stop. Our testers could not achieve this and had to take frequent short breaks. To begin with, you will probably need to break your daily half-hour stint into about three 10 minute sessions. In fact, this is advisable to help you do the exercises briskly without flagging at the end. The reason for circling the rope backwards is that, done this way, skipping is particularly effective for firming the muscles at the back of the arms, and also in giving a lift to the bosom by strengthening the muscles supporting it.

Waist-slimming skip

As well as burning up calories at the top rate, this skipping variation is designed particularly to pull in and firm slack muscles around the waist and in the 'spare-tyre' waist-to-bosom area. It is also very effective for the upper-arm flab problem. Start with six simple backward skips. Then swing both arms to the left, outstretched at shoulder level, twisting your body towards them from the waist. Now swirl the skipping rope round in the air in backwards circles as you jump up and down (just as if you were skipping) five times. Now six simple skips again, and then, arms outstretched to the right, repeat the skipping rope swirl in that direction. Make sure that you twist from the waist and that your hips are facing forwards when you do the sideways movement.
▼

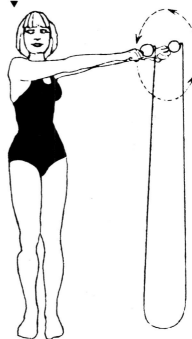

◄ Cross-over skip

If you do the simple backwards skip but cross your arms over your chest and cross the ropes on alternate jumps you make the exercise slightly more energetic — and even more beneficial for calorie-burn-up. (If you have not skipped for years you might find this difficult at first.) Unlike the other exercises, this exercise works another group of muscles supporting the bosom and across the shoulders. Therefore a good idea would be to alternate it with sessions of simple backwards skips.

The top calorie burners

How tired an activity makes you feel is often not a real indication, alas, of its effectiveness as an aid to weight control. Thus you can feel exhausted after tackling such everyday household tasks as a big pile of ironing or by typing for a long time but, because only limited arm movement is involved, the calorie output may well disappoint you. Apart from tasks around the house like polishing silver, window cleaning or scrubbing floors, where small movements are performed vigorously, it is the amount of walking around and general body movement that really determine how many calories you burn up at home. Cooking, for instance, tends to burn up slightly more calories than preparing vegetables because it normally involves more movement around the kitchen. Vacuum-cleaning tends to burn up more calories than cooking because of walking to and fro with the vacuum cleaner. The woman who lives in a small, well-designed home and has all the electrical equipment and gadgets she needs consequently does little physical work and, unless she exercises regularly or has a demanding job, may well burn up few extra calories.

Likewise, a hard day of mental work does not burn up a lot of calories as the brain uses up only about one-fifth of a calorie a minute. And, as with some computers that use only fractionally more electric current when calculating than when idling, the busy brain uses little more energy than the idle brain. Medical experts tell us that the feeling of fatigue is partly a psychological and partly a nervous phenomenon. The brain cells get fatigued, causing a general feeling of tiredness. If we were called upon to sprint a mile, however, or to undertake any other physical task after a day's mental slog, we would perform just as efficiently as if we had spent the whole day watching television. Switching from mental to physical work often helps to refresh the tired brain.

The form of exercise you do to burn up extra calories is important. The yoga-type stretching exercises or arm-swings and toe-touches will do wonders for your muscle tone but will not necessarily burn up many calories. To increase calorie expenditure you have to move your body from point A to point B at speed. Fast walking, for example, uses up more calories than slow walking, and jogging or running will burn up almost twice as many calories as most speeds of walking.

To reach the ultimate speeds of calorie expenditure, you need to move your whole body quickly and then add another factor

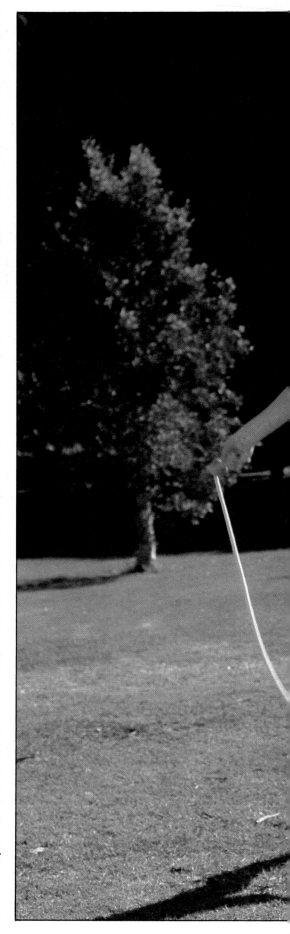

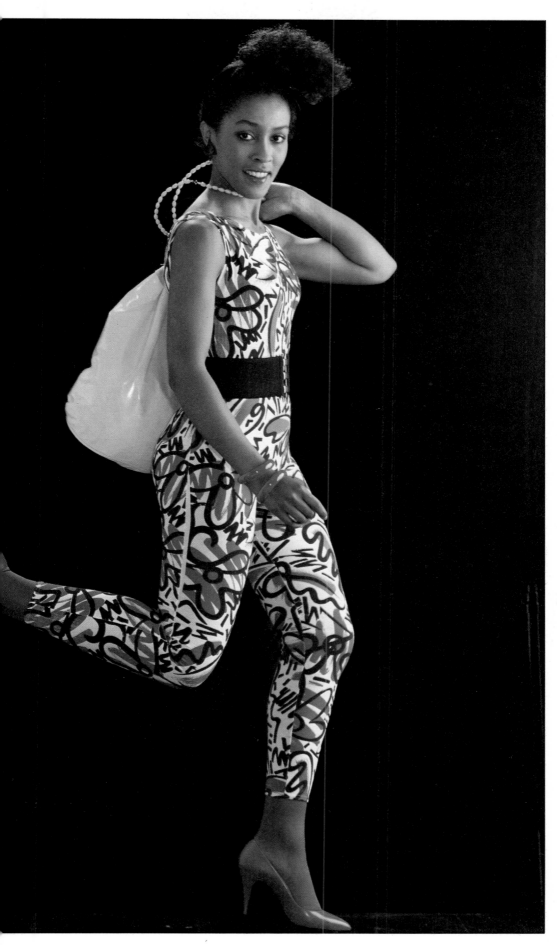

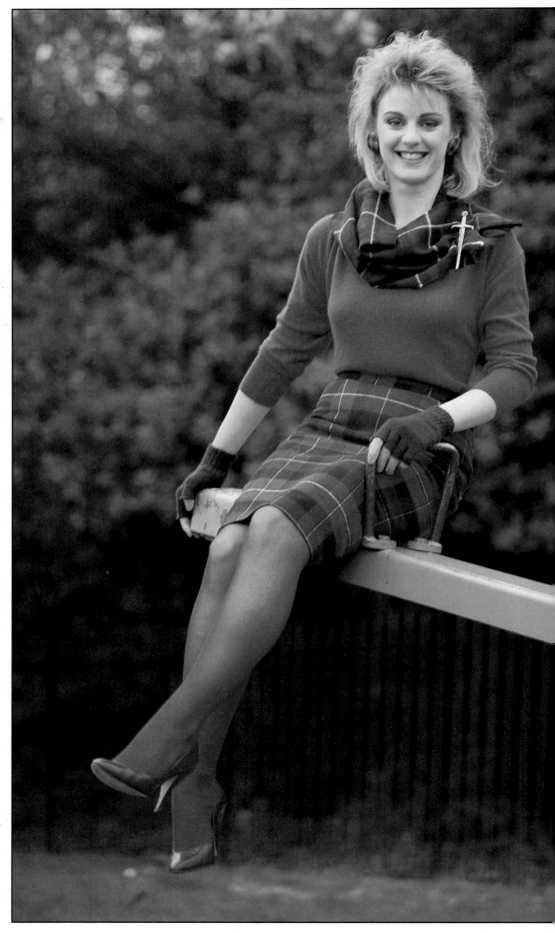

The trimming down of Tracey

'Farrell the Barrel'. That's what they called Tracey when she was an overweight child. At 13-years-old, she went on her first diet. She cut out sweets, stodgy puddings and visits to the chip shop, and it worked. Tracey managed to stay quite slim until she started going out with Derek when she was 17. After having a few drinks at a local pub, they regularly enjoyed going for feasts in an Indian or Chinese restaurant — and soon Tracey's weight was piling back on. Just over twelve months later, she had gained 19kg (3st). At 1.6m (5ft 3in) and weighing 76kg (12st), Tracey dreaded the summer. She could no longer hide behind dark, heavy, winter clothes, and she also suffered heat rashes and blisters that formed where her legs rubbed together. Her seaside holiday that year was a disaster. Despite the glorious sunshine, she spent most of her time huddled morosely in her deckchair, fully-clothed. Six months later, on New Year's Eve, Tracey was in despair as she tried on yet another awful outfit that she'd bought simply because it almost fitted her. And she made a New Year's Resolution to lose that ageing excess weight. She joined a slimming club and there she was put on a diet of 1,250 calories a day, with a target weight of 54kg (8st 7lb). Tracey went home that evening buzzing with excitement and determination. She lost weight at a steady average of 1kg (2lb) a week. Sometimes she ate more than her limit, but then she'd compensate with less the next day. Halfway through her diet, she bought a size twelve skirt and tried it on regularly. At first it wouldn't do up, then it fitted snugly . . . then it was too big! Four months after joining her club, she reached target weight. The next summer holiday Tracey took was very different from the previous year. This time she swam and leapt about in shorts and skimpy T-shirts. All things she could never have imagined herself doing when she was overweight.

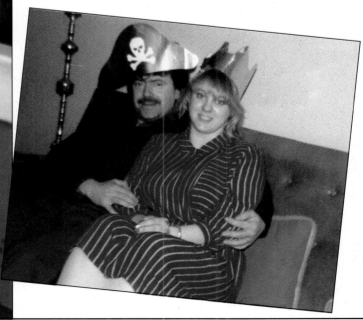

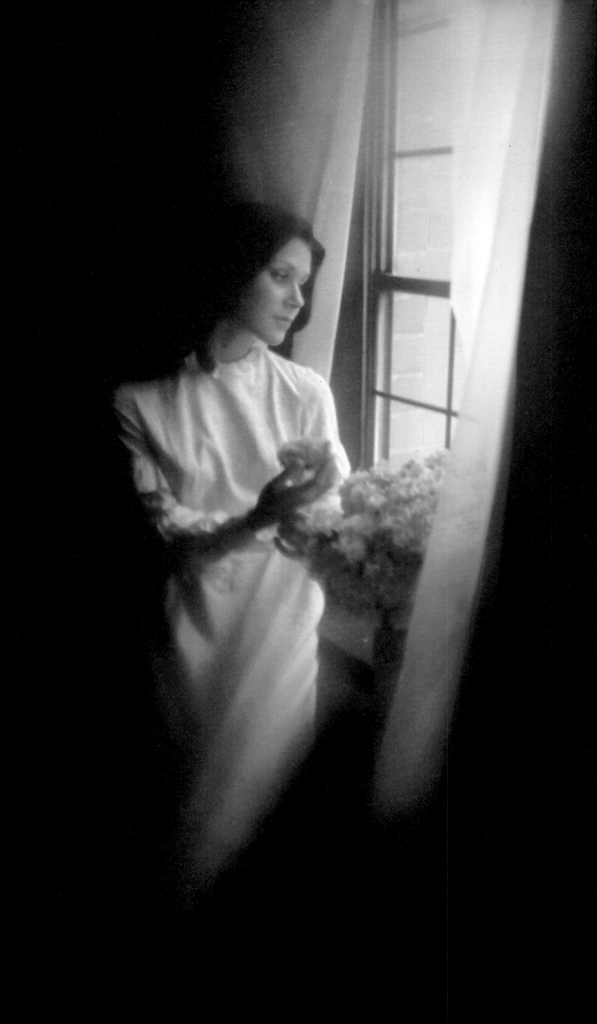

Strategy 2: Enjoy your food

This means every mouthful! Mindless eating is one of the slimmer's worst enemies. It's all too easy to grab sandwiches on the wing, eat quick snacks while your mind is on your work, or dig into biscuits and sweets while you're buried in a book or a good TV programme. But it is vitally important to your long-term success that *every* calorie you eat gives maximum physiological and psychological pleasure. The way to attain this is to be *aware* of what you are doing when you are eating, so that you enjoy and savour every mouthful. Lay your tray or table attractively. Sit down to eat. Eat slowly. Put your knife and fork down between bites. Have a favourite low-calorie drink with your meal, if you like, and savour it as you sip it. Enjoy snacks in the same way. Sit down with your cup of coffee. If you have counted a biscuit or cake in with your diet calories, enjoy every little bit. If you can learn to do this, you will be giving your diet resolution the right kind of psychological boost. There is a great deal of evidence to show that, when you are fully aware of what you are eating and enjoying the flavours and textures of your foods, you are satisfied with a smaller quantity. Many successful slimmers have found that, by eliminating mindless eating, they effortlessly cut their calorie intake quite considerably.

Strategy 3: Plan for temptation

No human being can resist the temptation to eat delicious foods and unnecessary calories *every* single day of *every* month of *every* year. There is always going to be temptation in the form of birthdays, parties and celebrations. Somebody will open a box of chocolates; somebody else will serve a scrumptious cake. When these occasions

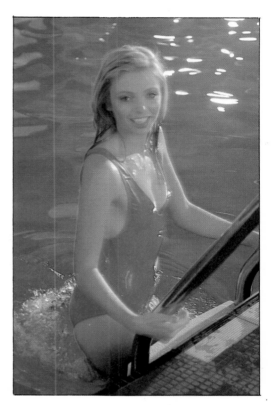

Swimming is not only one of the best forms of exercise, it can also help to take your mind off food and increase your confidence about your body image.

happen, you would be superhuman if you could say 'No' every time.

So, as far as you can, plan for them. If there is a special occasion in the offing, you can still enjoy it. If you are serious about shedding your surplus weight, you can either cut down on calories for a day or two beforehand, so that you have extra 'in the bank' to spend on champagne and wedding

Time: start–finish	Physical stance	Where and with whom	Mood	How hungry (scale 0–5)	Food and amount	Calories
7.45–8.00 a.m.	Standing	Alone in kitchen, making family breakfast	Tired	1	2 cups of tea with milk and 10ml (2 level teaspoons) sugar ·	75
8.00–8.20 a.m.	Sitting	At family breakfast	Neutral	1	2 small slices toast with 15g (½oz) butter and 10ml (2 teaspoons) honey	265
8.40–9.00 a.m.	Moving to clear table	Kitchen, alone	A bit tense	0	10ml (2 teaspoons) honey to finish pot; 1 cup of tea with milk and 5ml (1 teaspoon) sugar	80

cake or whatever; or you can make up for the extra calorie intake by cutting down afterwards. Either way will work because what counts is your total calorie consumption over, say, a period of one week. It really doesn't matter if you eat more calories than your diet permits on one day and less on another. If, at the end of the week, you have stayed within your total dieting calorie allowance, you're doing fine, and will continue to shed surplus weight.

There are also going to be times when you have an *unexpected* encounter with temptation and you will perhaps lose control. Maybe it's the whiff of freshly-baked bread or the sight of chocolate at the checkout that causes the downfall. Forgive yourself for your slip, and then be extra careful with your calorie intake for a couple of days to get the balance right again.

However, next time an unplanned temptation comes your way, do remember the strategy of eating slowly and *enjoying* every mouthful. Guilt has a remarkable way of ruining the taste buds, and leaving nothing behind but a feeling of self-reproach! If you can say to yourself: 'All right, I'm giving in to temptation, but I'm going to make this a deliberate, *aware* act. I'm going to enjoy this food and savour every mouthful,' you will enjoy your unscheduled indulgence with relish and will be far less likely to eat too much. Of course, if you give into temptation every single day, you won't lose weight! But if occasionally you simply can't resist something, don't waste time blaming 'weak willpower' or being 'fed-up'. Just accept that you are human. And get back on to your weight-control diet immediately afterwards.

Strategy 4: Protect your willpower
Willpower is a fragile thing at the best of times and, tested repeatedly, it will finally break. So you'll have a much easier dieting campaign if you avoid putting your willpower continually to the test.

Try not to have any of your downfall foods (the foods you know you can't resist if they are around) on the premises, except in the limited quantities that you are incorporating into your diet. And *don't* have high-calorie snack items like nuts, sweets, biscuits and chocolate lying around 'for others to eat'. Ask your family to help your diet by buying their own snack foods, and not to leave them around or eat them in front of you. Remember, what you buy, you will eat. So, unless they are a planned part of your slimming programme, don't buy high-calorie 'treats' on *any* excuse. If you do, they are likely to haunt you until you throw away the last wrapper.

Make it more *difficult* for yourself to get at tempting foods. If you see left-over pie every time you open the fridge door, or your glance falls on jars full of currants and glacé cherries all the time, you are making things *unnecessarily* hard for yourself. Keep leftovers well-wrapped, preferably in boxes with lids on and put foods like currants in opaque containers behind closed doors.

Don't go shopping on an empty stomach. If you plan a foray to the supermarket after you have recently enjoyed a satisfying meal, the temptation to sabotage your diet is far less likely to rear its ugly head. If you are out socially, try to keep your distance from all the random foods on offer. Nuts, crisps and canapés are invariably very high in calories, and they are an invitation to 'mindless' eating if you're close by. If you have to fight your way to them across a crowded room, it is that much easier to save your diet and your weight-loss promises.

Strategy 5: Eliminate let-out clauses
Some hopeful slimmers are passionately resolved to keep to a reducing diet, provided they are able to make a number of exceptions. They say to themselves: 'I'll keep to my diet like a saint except when visitors come to call/I'm entertaining/I'm going out for a meal/I'm joining the family or friends for a celebration/I'm offered food by So-and-so, who will be offended if I don't eat it/I'm at a business lunch/I'm at a party/the food has been paid for and mustn't be wasted/I'm out with friends at a pub or the wine bar . . .'

If you seriously want to shed surplus weight, you can't allow yourself any kind of double-think, however unconscious. Sit down and write out a list of the situations in which you honestly consider it reasonable to deviate a little from your weight-loss programme. The aim is to make you aware of the diet let-out clauses which you *genuinely* feel apply to your circumstances, so that you can plan accordingly (see Strategy 3!) But, as you will realize if you think about it, if you embark on a slimming aim with a list even half as long as the one above, you may have little hope of success. Firmly eliminate all but the one or two let-outs that are truly important to you.

Strategy 6: Have other things to do
Many an idle snack is eaten out of boredom, and much uncontrolled eating is triggered off by a blue mood. But if you are trying to control our weight, it is best not to deal with negative moods and frustrations by putting extra calories into your mouth. The good feeling lasts a very short time. The bad feel-

ings can last long enough to wreak destruction on dieting resolutions. What can you do instead? If your only way to alleviate tedium, gloom or misery is to eat, it could be imperative for your long-term well-being and morale to find more positive and constructive activities to engage in.

Doing something positive instead of eating isn't easy if you are feeling negative. But it is infinitely rewarding, both in terms of your slimming programme and in terms of your emotional well-being and self-confidence. There is no question that you will feel much better about yourself and about life in general if you anticipate boredom, loneliness or anger — or any other negative state of mind that makes you want to eat — by having some other activity planned which you are ready to get on with.

When a bad mood strikes, force yourself to break the negative spell with *some* activity. Have a couple of lists ready, one headed 'Work: Chores I'd like to get done'; the other entitled 'Fun: Things I like doing'.

'Work' includes items like sewing on buttons, clearing out drawers, sorting out clothes or weeding flowerbeds. 'Fun' includes pleasant activities that have no visible rewards but which make you feel good while you are doing them — such as tackling a crossword puzzle, having a scented bath, arranging flowers, reading a good book, or walking through the park.

Sort your lists out into tasks or pastimes that take five minutes, ten minutes, half an hour, and so on. Then, next time a blue mood strikes, you will be ready for it. When you feel an impulse to head towards the kitchen for some kind of comfort-eating, pick up the lists and do one of the chores or pastimes *first*.

If, when you've cleared out the drawer, had the bath, or whatever, you still feel an overwhelming urge to eat, have a *little* of the food you crave . . . and *enjoy* it. Sit down and eat it slowly. Savour it. Know what you are doing.

Doing something positive with your time instead of taking the easy way out will foster a sense of confidence and well-being that can definitely only benefit your slimming campaign.

Losing body hang-ups

There has been a vast amount of serious scientific research into ordinary people's sex lives, including in-depth confidential interviews with many thousands of men and women. Yet studies comparing the intimate lives of overweight and slim women have shown a marked similarity in the sexual behaviour of both groups. Indeed, surplus weight, in itself, emerges as no handicap to a happy and fulfilled sex life.

These findings, however, can be of little comfort to the woman plagued by the problem of excess weight. But if you are unhappy because of the way your feelings about your shape are affecting your relationships, it is important to get this whole issue into perspective. To embark on a weight-loss programme for the sake or your confidence and your health is unquestionably desirable; but it is also important for the self-conscious overweight woman to realize that a 'perfect' slim figure is not the only acceptable shape she need have in order to achieve happiness, success and sexual fulfilment. The real world is full of women whose figures by so-called 'ideal' standards are too plump, too thin, too short or too tall. Yet these women are happily attractive to their men, and just as successful in every sphere of life as they want to be.

Statistically, the marriage rate is exactly the same for overweight women as it is for slim ones – another confirmation that men aren't looking for 'perfection' in their partners. They are no different from women in being attracted to a partner who is outgoing and friendly, who cares about herself, and who is not afraid of her body, or ashamed of it. A woman, in other words, who has learned not to let secret hang-ups about her size or any other real or imagined body 'flaw' come between her and the world she lives in.

All of us, when we first meet a person, make an instantaneous judgment about whether this is someone we want to approach or move away from. Unconsciously, we are reacting to the secret signals that person is sending out — the signs that tell us whether he or she feels good about life, and is ready to be interested and enjoy the moment we're sharing.

A woman who does not consider herself to be appealing will signal this to others. If she suffers from low self-esteem, it can have a marked and unfortunate effect on her behaviour. She may have allowed her own low opinion of herself to influence the way she dresses and presents herself to the world, so that she looks more dowdy and depressed than she realizes. Depending on her temperament, she may find an apathetic and apparently 'stand-offish' reaction to others her easiest form of self-protection. Or she may strike a self-protective 'good pal, one of the boys' pose in order to indicate that she is not 'competing' as a sexually attractive woman.

All aspects of appearance, including body weight, do play a major part in initial attraction between people — but *only* initially. What count in the long term are warmth, interest and vitality — qualities that can be cultivated and are irresistible to everyone — no matter what shape they come in.

Pauline turns into a knock-out!

Pauline Hemming had always been fat and had come to terms with it. In fact, she thought it was her only option. She grew up with comments like: 'It's in your nature to be well-built' and 'You wouldn't be *you* if you were any thinner'. Despite rolls of fat that wobbled whenever she moved, Pauline still fooled herself that her size had nothing to do with the pie, chips, crisps and six or seven bars of chocolate she consumed every day, and she refused to admit that her weight was a major problem. After all, she and Dennis had been together for fourteen years. They'd made a lovely home together. She had a good job. So who cared about weight? But, deep-down inside, she knew it was the main reason why they had never married. Who wants to be a hugely heavyweight bride? The wedding could wait. Over the years, since her weight had soared from its 'normal' 95.5kg (15st) to 124kg (19½st), she had been getting more difficult to live with. Dennis's favourite joke was that, as a fireman, he'd never be first up any ladder to rescue her — he'd be too afraid of risking injury from carrying such an abnormal load! As Pauline's confidence sank lower and lower, every innocent comment by Dennis would stab her like a knife. They were gradually turning into two very unhappy people. There were blush-making incidents to make her working life miserable, too. If a girl of normal weight happens to break her office chair, everyone assumes it is the chair's fault. When the back of Pauline's swivel chair snapped right off, the office administrator didn't hesitate to blame *her*. Finally, it was the discovery that, at 1.73m (5ft 8in), she weighed 19kg (3st) more than 1.90m (6ft 3in) boxing star Frank Bruno that shocked Pauline into slimming. It took a year for her to reach her target weight of 62kg (9st 10lb). It wasn't sunshine all the way, but she never let the odd slip stop her from getting right back on course. And becoming slim gave Pauline the confidence to switch to an even better job, to discover a far more rewarding lifestyle, and to enter and win *Slimming Magazine's* UK Slimmer of the Year contest.

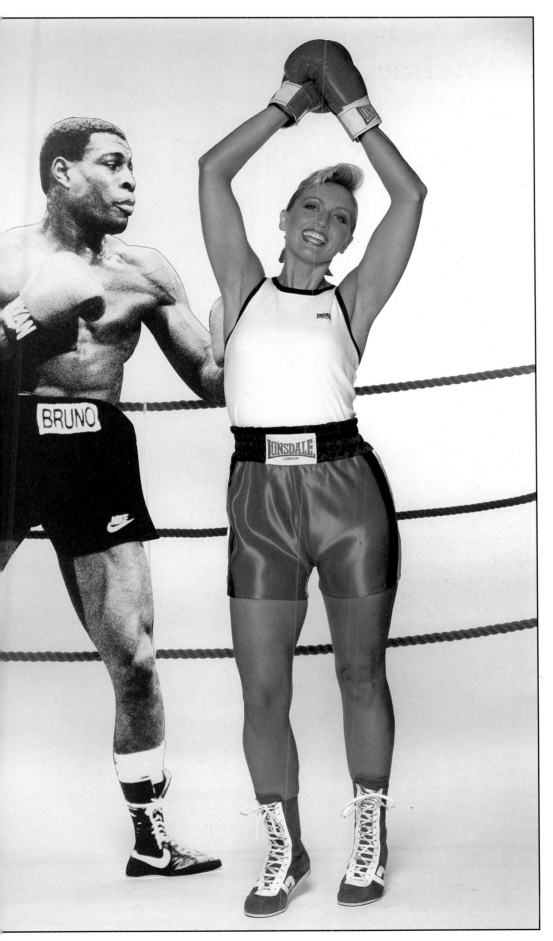

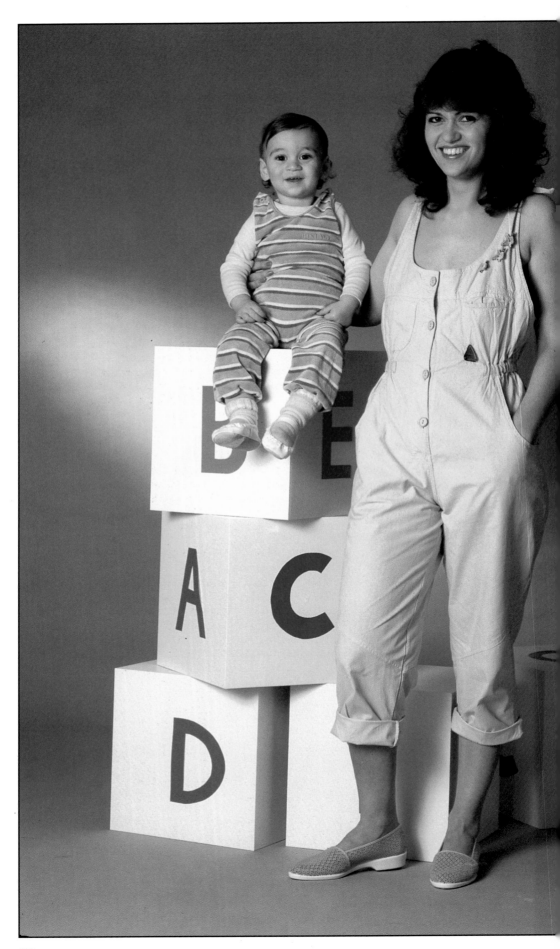

The 'pudding' who became a delicious 'soufflé'

Marie-Lise had been a tiny size 10 when she came to England from France to study. Then she met and married Ron. Within seven short months she had managed to eat her way up to a huge size 18. As she counted on having a baby as soon as she could, it didn't seem worth getting a job, so she became a full-time housewife. She spent her days sitting around the house reading romantic novels and cooking meals. To pass the time, she ate and, the more she ate, the bigger her appetite grew. Soon, out of boredom, she was eating whether she was hungry or not. As she got fatter, she lost her confidence and found she couldn't mix with other people. She looked and felt like an old woman, even though she was only 24-years-old. Then, one Christmas, on a visit to her family in France, Marie-Lise had to face the truth. Her 10-year-old nephew, Jean-Phillippe, decided to try out his new instant camera. When he revealed the results, Marie-Lise was horrified. Her face and neck looked swollen and enormous, and she had bulges everywhere. She took a really good look at herself and hated what she saw, then climbed on the scales for the first time in months. At 78.2kg (12st 4lb) she knew she had to lose weight, yet she still badly wanted a baby. Her brother took pity on her and arranged for her to see a gynaecologist. The gynaecologist told her firmly that being fat wouldn't make her pregnant — if anything, it would hinder conception. Marie-Lise started to diet, but before reaching her ideal weight, she discovered that the longed-for baby was on its way! A month after Michael was born, she went out and bought *Slimming Magazine*. Now she wanted to be slim so that Michael would grow up proud of her and have a mother who could run about and play with him. She put a size-10 skirt on a hanger outside her wardrobe and tried it on every day, determined that she was going to get into it. The surplus weight steadily went away. Within two months, she was at her target 52kg (8st 3lb) and, as she shed her weight, she shed her hang-ups. Marie-Lise felt wonderful and her bubbly personality bloomed again.

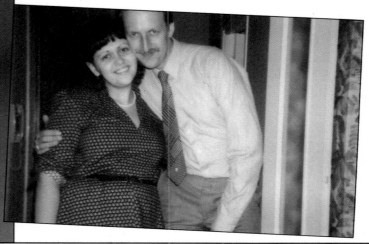

Rosemary's dream comes true

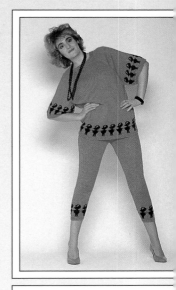

Rosemary Partridge wallowed for years in a passion for chocolate, and the result was to find herself miserable and massive. She was a 1.78m (5ft 10in) mountain weighing 79.5kg (12½st). The worst thing about her surplus 13kg (2st) was that it gave her a very embarrassing shape. Her enormous stomach made her look as if she was about to have a baby. When, at 18, she married for the first time, she soon became used to people thinking she was pregnant. When Rosemary's marriage broke up, she couldn't be bothered to prepare meals and she nibbled instead, feeding herself with a never-ending stream of sweets and calorie-filled snacks. It was after her second marriage, when people again started hinting that she looked pregnant, that Rosemary knew she was going to have to do something about her 107cm (42in) bust and her 114cm (45in) hips. Deciding, at last, to exert some honest effort, Rosemary started slimming. Basically, her diet included much the same kind of food that most families enjoy. Her husband had also been married before and she now had three children to cook for, as well. It was mainly a matter of making wiser choices, taking smaller portions and learning how to assess calorie values so that they became second nature to her. When Rosemary stood on the scales after her first week's dieting, she couldn't believe her eyes. She had lost 3.5kg (8lb). At the end of the second week, another 2.5kg (6lb) had been slimmed away. Within a fortnight, a whole 6kg (1st) of surplus weight had disappeared. In ten weeks, after having been fat for 20 years, she had reached target weight, and her shape had undergone an amazing transformation. No more stomach bulge, a slender waist, a tiny bottom, and legs that seemed to have stretched to look longer and slimmer. This was how Rosemary had dreamed of looking since she was a child. Now, at 25 years of age, her ambition had finally been achieved.

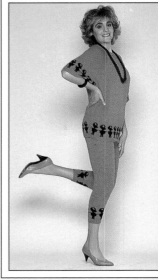

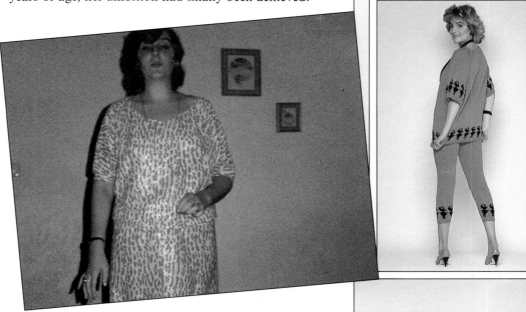

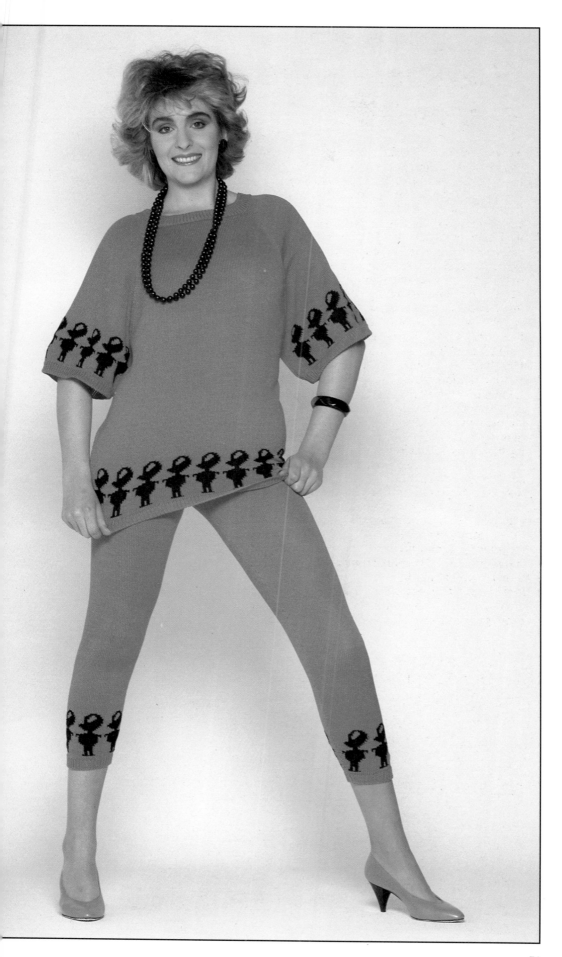

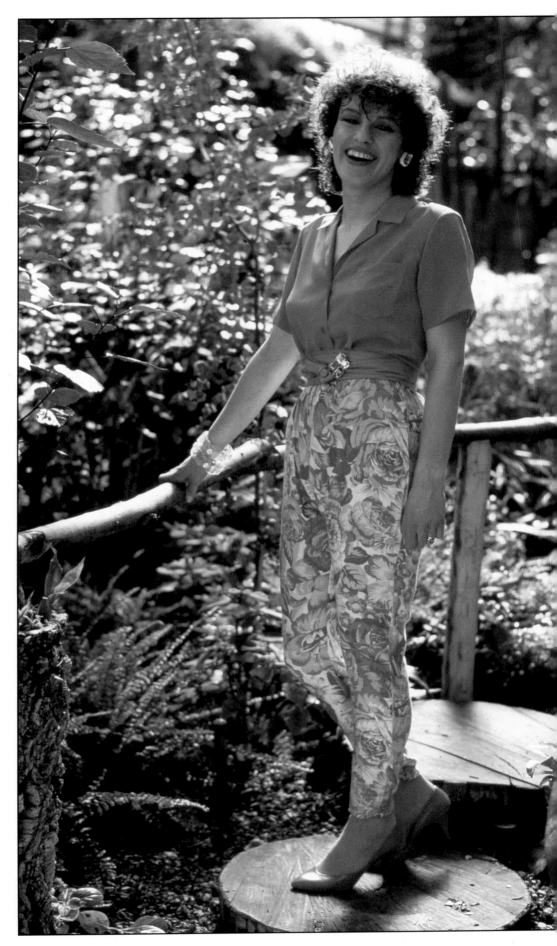

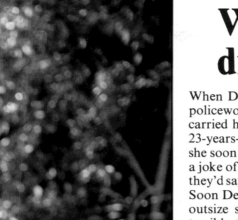

What 12 months did for Debbie

When Debbie Cockcroft went to college to train to be a policewoman, she was already hefty. But despite this, she carried her weight well and loved smart clothes. She was 23-years-old when she married Mark. At 1.65m (5ft 5in), she soon weighed 82.6kg (13st). At work, her friends made a joke of her ever-increasing flab. 'Lead the way, Big Girl,' they'd say when trouble broke out, 'we're right behind you!' Soon Debbie had to limit clothes-shopping expeditions to outsize shops, and wearing a uniform in size-24 was a terrible torment. Spurred on by a colleague, she decided to go along to her local slimming club. It was friendly, relaxed and cheerful. But it wasn't nice to see the scales say 103kg (16st 3lb), or to learn that her target weight would be 57.5kg (9st). The first week, she lost 3kg (6lb), then her weekly weight loss settled down to a regular 1–1.5kg (2–3lbs) a week. In twelve months, she had lost 45.5kg (100lb). The only people who weren't overly-delighted with Debbie's transformation were the folks in the police stores. The first time she visited them, slopping around inside her cavernous size-24 uniform and asking for a smaller swap, they thought it was hilarious. Then, when she went back to trade in her swap, they didn't laugh quite so loudly. They looked positively miffed when she reappeared asking for a third exchange. And it was 'Not you again!' when finally she applied for her size-12. At one stage during Operation Countdown, Debbie got a bit worried. Would losing bulk make her a less effective policewoman and more of a pushover for villains? She needn't have worried. What she lost in weight, she more than gained in extra energy, fitness, confidence and, perhaps, diplomacy. Now, when they meet a tricky character, her colleagues often seek her out to defuse the situation. 'Go on, Debbie,' they'll say, 'use your charm.'

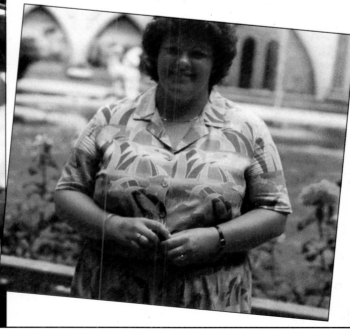

When you can see precisely one calorie — as you can 45 times in the foods pictured on these pages — it is surprising how much easier it becomes to assess the number of calories you are eating. So here's looking at you, calorie...

One calorie

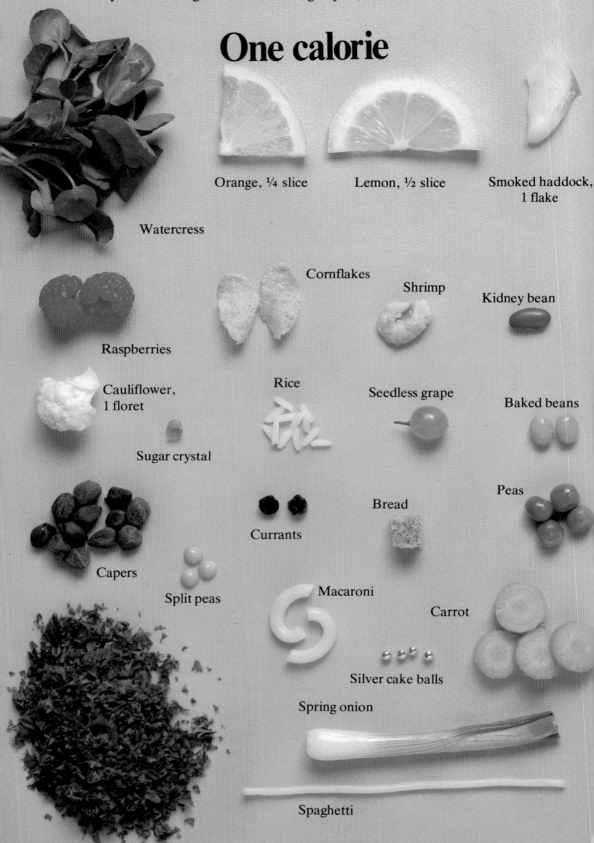

Orange, ¼ slice

Lemon, ½ slice

Smoked haddock, 1 flake

Watercress

Cornflakes

Shrimp

Kidney bean

Raspberries

Cauliflower, 1 floret

Rice

Seedless grape

Baked beans

Sugar crystal

Peas

Capers

Currants

Bread

Split peas

Macaroni

Carrot

Silver cake balls

Spring onion

Spaghetti

Parsley

CHAPTER 6

Calories on view

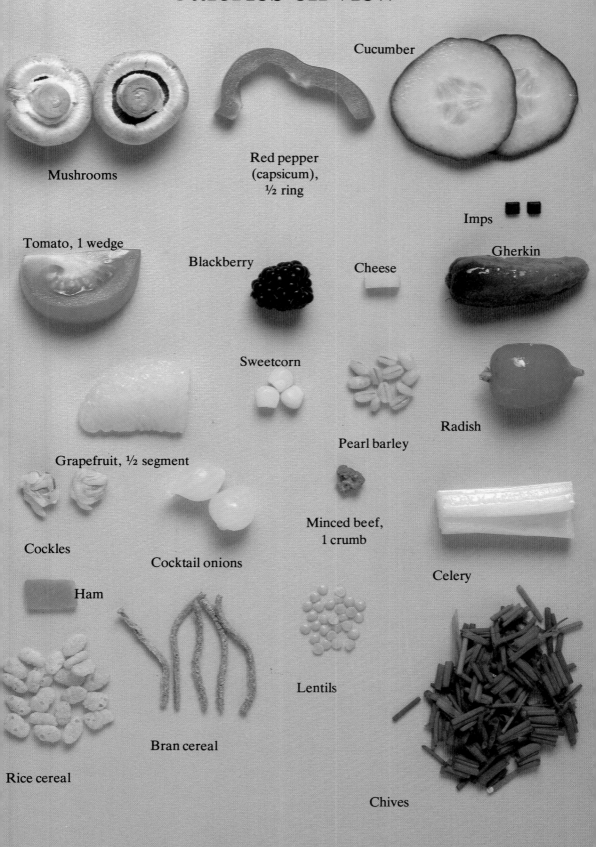

Mushrooms

Red pepper
(capsicum),
½ ring

Cucumber

Imps

Tomato, 1 wedge

Blackberry

Cheese

Gherkin

Sweetcorn

Pearl barley

Radish

Grapefruit, ½ segment

Cockles

Cocktail onions

Minced beef,
1 crumb

Celery

Ham

Lentils

Bran cereal

Chives

Rice cereal

The nothing foods

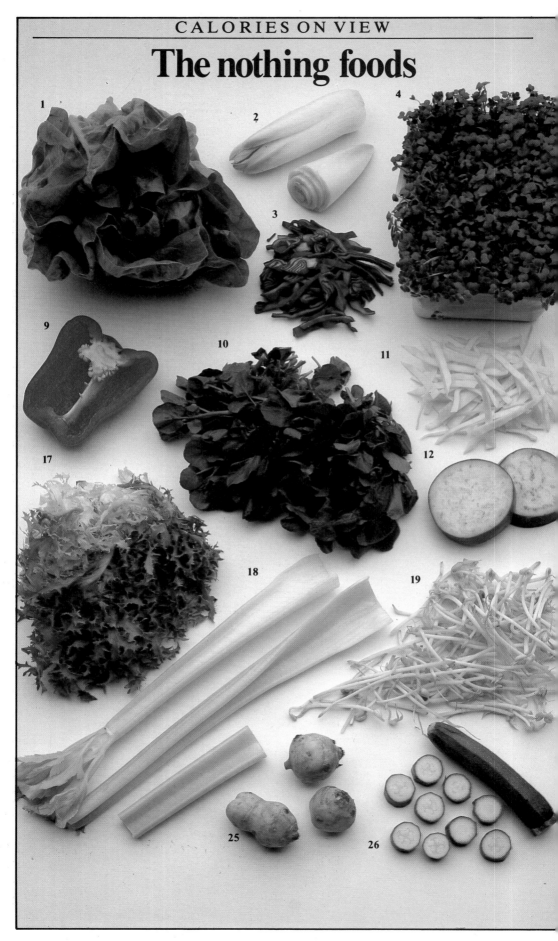

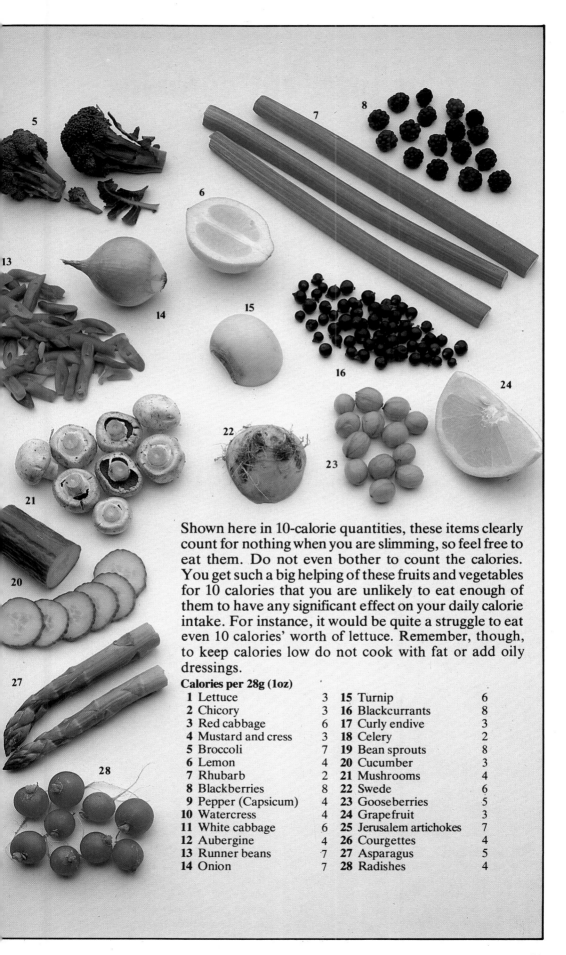

Shown here in 10-calorie quantities, these items clearly count for nothing when you are slimming, so feel free to eat them. Do not even bother to count the calories. You get such a big helping of these fruits and vegetables for 10 calories that you are unlikely to eat enough of them to have any significant effect on your daily calorie intake. For instance, it would be quite a struggle to eat even 10 calories' worth of lettuce. Remember, though, to keep calories low do not cook with fat or add oily dressings.

Calories per 28g (1oz)

1 Lettuce	3	15 Turnip	6
2 Chicory	3	16 Blackcurrants	8
3 Red cabbage	6	17 Curly endive	3
4 Mustard and cress	3	18 Celery	2
5 Broccoli	7	19 Bean sprouts	8
6 Lemon	4	20 Cucumber	3
7 Rhubarb	2	21 Mushrooms	4
8 Blackberries	8	22 Swede	6
9 Pepper (Capsicum)	4	23 Gooseberries	5
10 Watercress	4	24 Grapefruit	3
11 White cabbage	6	25 Jerusalem artichokes	7
12 Aubergine	4	26 Courgettes	4
13 Runner beans	7	27 Asparagus	5
14 Onion	7	28 Radishes	4

Cut fats, cut calories

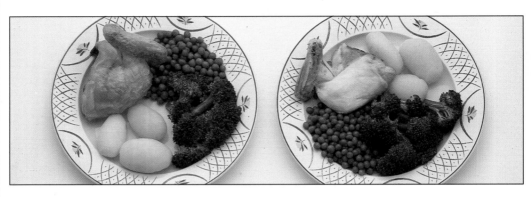

Roast chicken dinner

530 calories: 7½ fat units
All the fat here comes from the chicken. The 115g (4oz) boiled potatoes, 75g (3oz) peas and 75g (3oz) broccoli are fatless and contribute just 165 calories to this plateful.

355 calories: 2 fat units
When the chicken has been roasted, remove and discard the skin. You will automatically almost halve the calories of this wing quarter — down from 365 calories to 190.

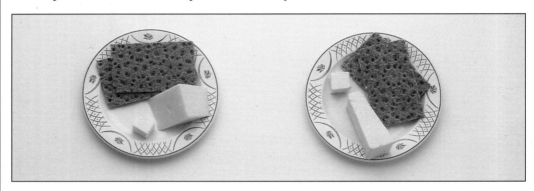

Crispbreads & cheese

340 calories: 9 fat units
Spread a couple of crispbreads with 7g (¼oz) butter and top with 50g (2oz) Cheddar cheese and your little snack costs pretty high.

225 calories: 4 fat units
Swap butter for low-fat spread and Cheddar cheese for a reduced-fat hard cheese and calories plus fat are cut considerably.

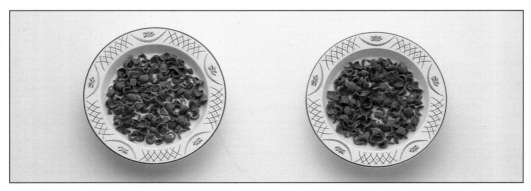

Cereal and milk

225 calories: 2½ fat units
This 40g (1½oz) bran cereal is served with 150ml (¼ pint) whole milk. If you also drink 275ml (½ pint) milk in drinks during the day, that is another 190 calories and 4 fat units.

180 calories: ½ fat unit
Serve the cereal with 150ml (¼ pint) skimmed milk and the calorie and fat content will come down. A daily 275ml (½ pint) skimmed milk would cost 100 calories but no fat.

You may not need to reduce the size of your meal to reduce your calorie intake. Often a simple swap from a high fat ingredient to a lower fat one does the trick. Here are some examples.

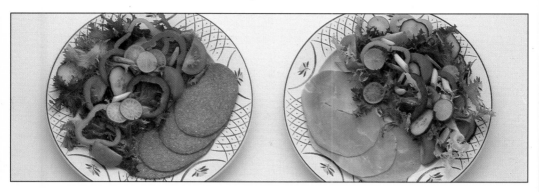

Cold meat salad

285 calories: 9 fat units
The only reason calories remain fairly reasonable for this salad is that the 50g (2oz) salami is served with very-low-calorie fatless salad vegetables.

120 calories: 1 fat unit
Choose lean cooked ham — cutting off any visible fat — instead of fatty salami and the calories in your salad will be more than halved.

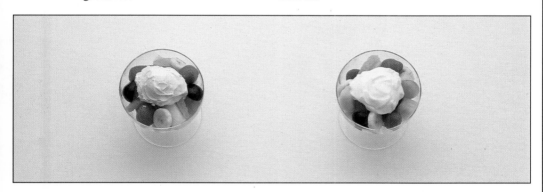

Fruit and topping

370 calories: 9½ fat units
Top a mixed fresh fruit salad with 50g (2oz) double cream and you'll add 255 calories to your dessert.

145 calories: ½ fat unit
Use 50g (2oz) low-fat natural yogurt as a topping and the calorie and fat difference is enormous.

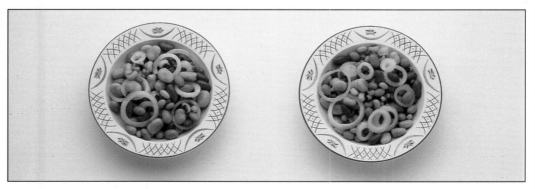

Dressed salad

530 calories: 12 fat units
A salad made with 225g (8oz) mixed boiled beans has just ½ fat unit – the remainder of fat here comes from the almost invisible 45ml (3 tablespoons) French dressing.

315 calories: ½ fat unit
Here is exactly the same amount of beans, but this time they are tossed in oil-free French dressing. The result is a massive reduction in fat and 215 fewer calories.

Calories by the spoonful

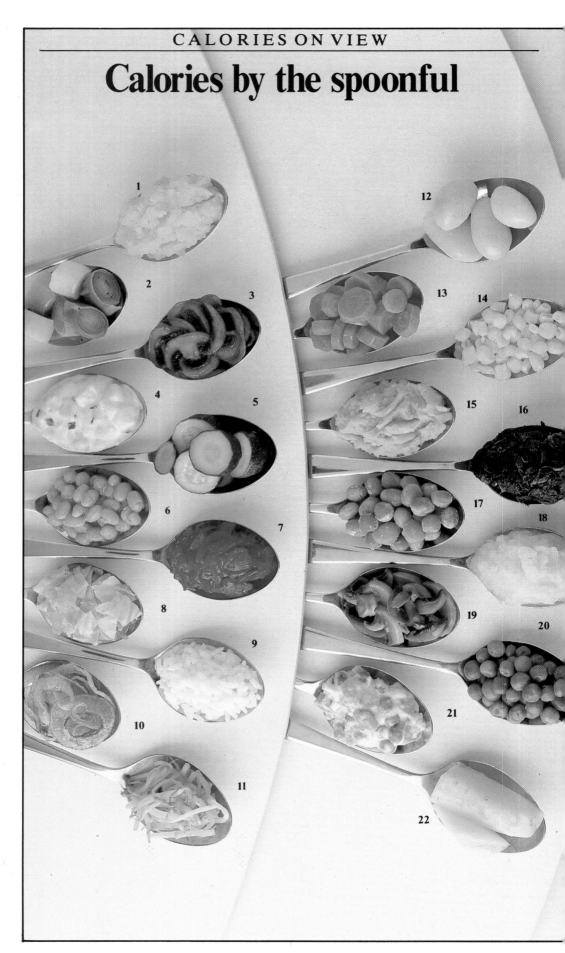

Spooning out vegetables to accompany meat and fish dishes is easy if you know their calorie values by the spoonful. Our at-a-glance picture guide shows you the number of calories per rounded tablespoon of some common foods.

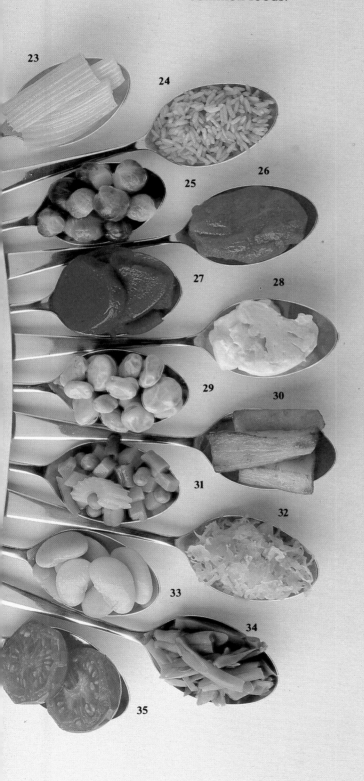

1	Swede, mashed	8
2	Leeks, boiled	7
3	Mushrooms, fried	40
4	Potato salad, canned	50
5	Courgettes	3
6	Baked beans	20
7	Pickled cabbage	3
8	Cabbage	2
9	Rice, boiled	20
10	Onions, fried	25
11	Bean sprouts, boiled	3
12	New potatoes	25
13	Carrots	5
14	Sweetcorn	20
15	Pease pudding	65
16	Spinach	10
17	Dried peas	30
18	Turnip, mashed	4
19	Mushrooms, stewed	2
20	Peas	15
21	Vegetable salad	50
22	Parsnips, boiled	16
23	Celery, braised	1
24	Rice, fried	70
25	Brussels sprouts	6
26	Tomato, canned	5
27	Beetroot, pickled	10
28	Cauliflower in white sauce	25
29	Broad beans	15
30	Parsnips, roast	30
31	Mixed vegetables	11
32	Sauerkraut	4
33	Butter beans	23
34	Runner beans	5
35	Tomato, fried	35

Calories by the carton

Frosted cornflakes
100 calories

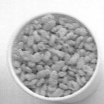
Rice cereal
65 calories

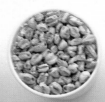
Puffed wheat cereal
40 calories

Special K
90 calories

Cornflakes
90 calories

Muesli
305 calories

**Porridge
made with water**
65 calories

**Crunchy oat and
nut cereal** 320 calories

Bran cereal
130 calories

Cracklin'bran
190 calories

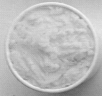
Potato, mashed
185 calories

Shredded cabbage, raw
10 calories

**Butter beans,
cooked**
125 calories

**Mashed swede
(no butter)**
30 calories

Creamed corn
155 calories

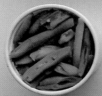
**Runner beans,
boiled** 25 calories

Broad beans, boiled
120 calories

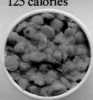
Mushy peas
145 calories

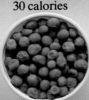
Frozen peas, boiled
55 calories

**Processed peas
canned**
105 calories

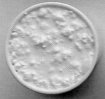
**Cottage cheese,per
113g (4oz) carton**
110 calories

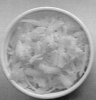
**Grated Cheddar
cheese** 245 calories

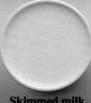
Skimmed milk
60 calories

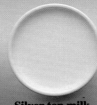
Silver top milk
110 calories

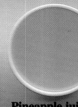
Pineapple juice
90 calories

White rice, boiled
130 calories

White spaghetti, boiled 130 calories

Keep an empty 115g (4oz) cottage cheese carton handy and say goodbye to guesswork. Just look at how many everyday foods can be calorie-counted in this way without getting out the scales. Measuring non-liquids, all calories are for loosely-packed cartons.

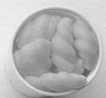

Pasta shells, boiled
135 calories

Brown spaghetti, boiled
95 calories

Brown rice, boiled
125 calories

Brown macaroni, boiled
95 calories

Sweetcorn kernels
75 calories

Spaghetti in tomato sauce
100 calories

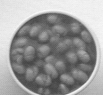

Baked beans in tomato sauce
115 calories

Rice pudding, canned
155 calories

Custard made with skimmed milk
130 calories

Frozen mixed vegetables, boiled
45 calories

Carrots, boiled
20 calories

Tomatoes, canned
20 calories

Stewed apple (no sugar)
70 calories

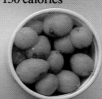

Stewed gooseberries, with sugar 70 calories

Orange juice, sweetened
35 calories

Orange juice, unsweetened
55 calories

Apple juice
60 calories

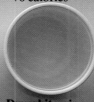

Dry white wine
115 calories

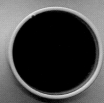

Red wine
120 calories

Fill up with fibre

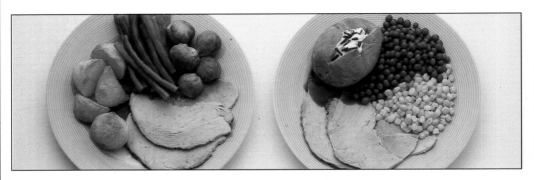

Roast dinner

495 calories: 9.6g fibre

Accompanying 75g (3oz) lean roast leg of pork (no fibre) are 175g (6oz) roast potatoes, 75g (3oz) Brussels sprouts, 115g (4oz) green beans and 30ml (2 tablespoons) fat-free gravy.

485 calories: 19.4g fibre

Higher fibre vegetables will more than double your meal's fibre content. Here the pork is served with 200g (7oz) potato, baked and topped with a tablespoon yogurt, 100g (3½oz) sweetcorn and 115g (4oz) peas.

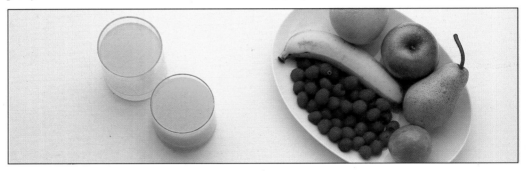

Fruit juice/fruit

230 calories: 0g fibre

Fruit juice may look super-healthy but it won't supply you with any fibre. And you could drink the unsweetened apple juice and orange juice shown here without feeling any fill-up satisfaction.

230 calories: 19.1g fibre

For the same number of calories, you'll get all this fruit, which will supply almost two-thirds of your daily recommended fibre intake.

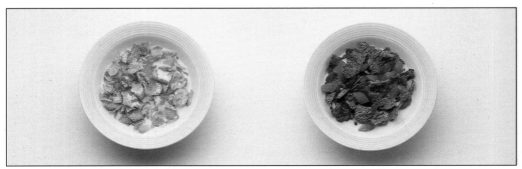

Cereal

210 calories: 0.4g fibre

This 25g (1oz) cornflakes is sprinkled with 20ml (2 rounded teaspoons) sugar and then topped with 115ml (4fl oz) skimmed milk.

210 calories: 12g fibre

Bran flakes have ten times more fibre than cornflakes. The 25g (1oz) dried apricots plus 15g (½oz) sultanas supply sweetness as well as lots more fibre than sugar.

Increasing your daily fibre intake may be just a matter of making the right sort of choices. All these meals are low enough in calories to fit into a day's dieting allowance. But the dish on the left is low in fibre, while the one on the right has at least a third of a day's 'ration'.

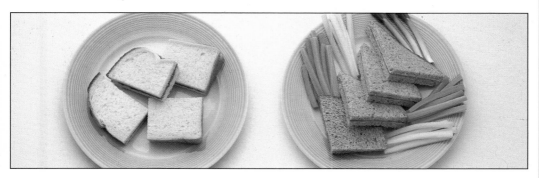

Sandwiches

380 calories: 2.3g fibre
This sandwich is made with two 40g (1½oz) slices white bread, 15g (½oz) low-fat spread and 35g (1¼oz) corned beef. All the fibre comes from the bread.

380 calories: 10.7g fibre
Wholemeal bread will supply 7.2g fibre. For a filling meal, the corned beef is reduced to 25g (1oz), then 50g (2oz) carrot, 1 stick celery and 3 spring onions added.

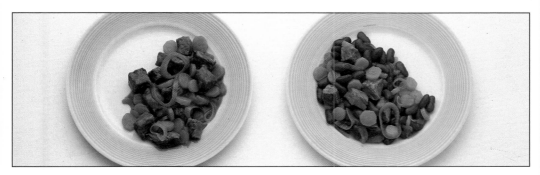

Casserole

205 calories: 2g fibre
All the fibre comes from the vegetables. To make this simple casserole 150g (5oz) lean braising steak is cooked with 25g (1oz) onions, 50g (2oz) carrots and ¼ stock cube mixed with water.

205 calories: 11.6g fibre
Here's how to increase fibre *and* get more for your calories. This casserole has less meat (50g/2oz) but more vegetables (115g/4oz red kidney beans and an extra 25g/1oz onion is added).

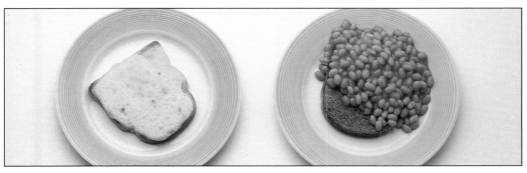

Toast meal

250 calories: 1.2g fibre
All the fibre in this meal comes from the 40g (1½oz) slice of white bread. It is topped with 35g (1¼ oz) Cheddar cheese.

250 calories: 20.1g fibre
There is more fibre in the 40g (1½oz) slice wholemeal bread. But a whole 16.5g fibre comes from 225g (7.9oz) can baked beans.

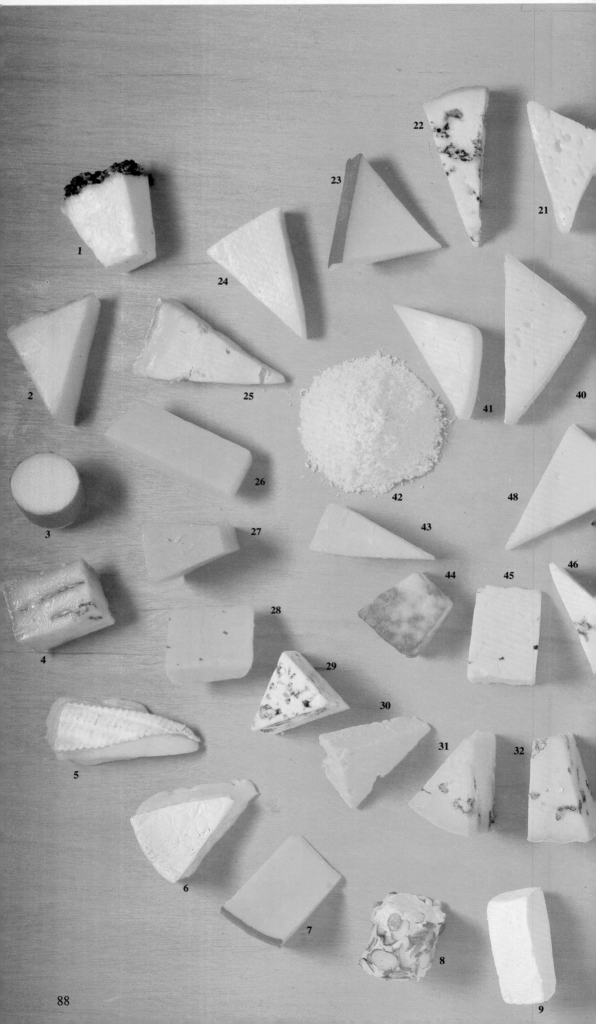

The cheese-eater's guide

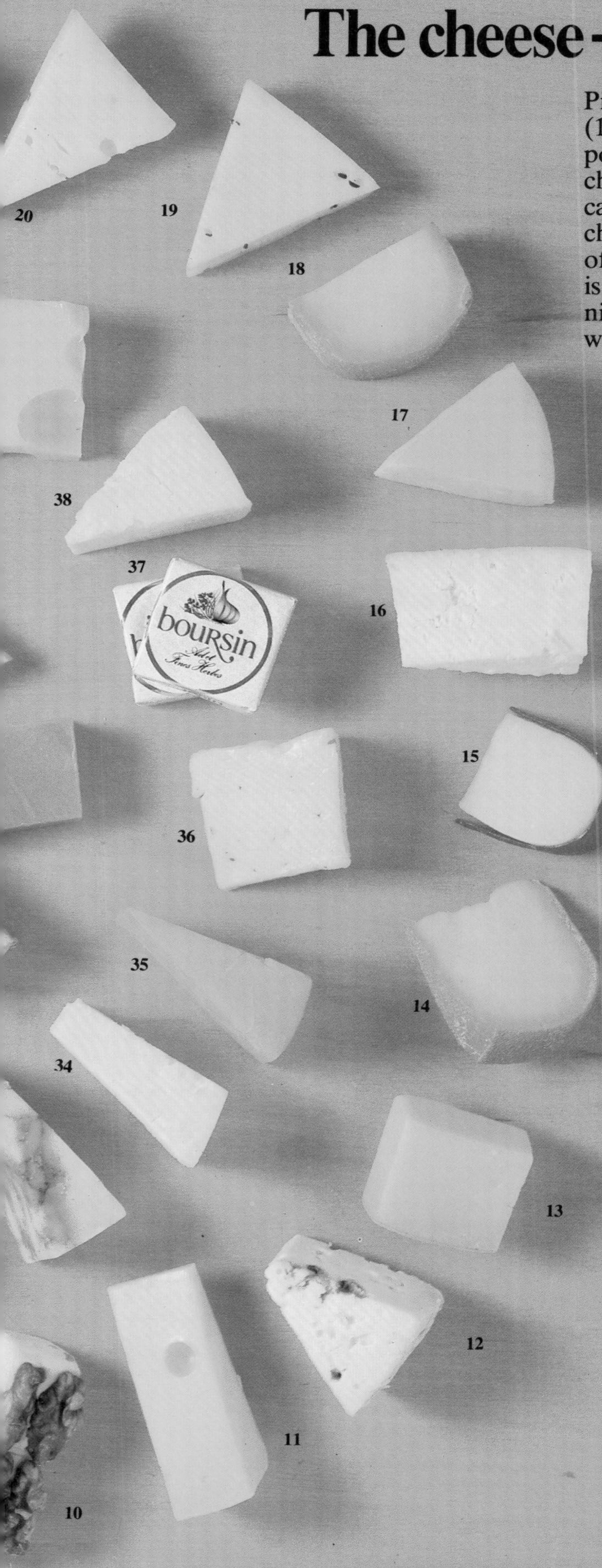

Pictured here are precise 28g (1oz) portions of a selection of popular English and continental cheeses, together with their calorie values. A small piece of cheese often provides quite a lot of calories and, as you can see, it is not a 'safe' food which can be nibbled between dieting meals without counting the calorie cost.

1	Tôme au raisin	94
2	Bel Paese	96
3	Austrian smoked	78
4	Bresse bleu	80
5	Brie	88
6	Camembert	88
7	Edam	90
8	Orangerulle	92
9	Philadelphia	90
10	Rambol with walnuts	117
11	Jarlsberg	95
12	Roquefort	88
13	Gouda	100
14	Port-Salut	94
15	Babybel	97
16	White Stilton	108
17	Bonbel	102
18	St Paulin	98
19	Danbo	97
20	Danish Mozzarella	98
21	Danish Esrom	90
22	Danish Mycella	100
23	Danish Elbo	97
24	Danish Samsoe	101
25	Dolcellata	100
26	Double Gloucester	105
27	Leicester	105
28	Cotswold	105
29	Danish blue	100
30	Cheshire	110
31	Blue Cheshire	124
32	Gorgonzola	112
33	Sage Derby	115
34	Lancashire	109
35	Orkney Claymore	111
36	Ilchester	112
37	Boursin	116
38	Wensleydale	115
39	Emmenthal	115
40	Danish Havarti	117
41	Caerphilly	120
42	Parmesan	118
43	Cheddar	120
44	Red Windsor	119
45	Cheviot	120
46	Blue Stilton	131
47	Norwegian Gjeost	133
48	Gruyère	117

boursin

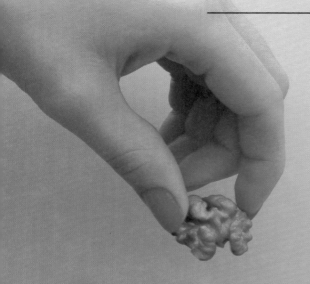

Piece of peanut brittle
50 calories

Walnut half
15 calories

Chocolate peanut
5 calories

Brazil nut
20 calories

Sugared almond
15 calories

Triangle of nut chocolate
30 calories

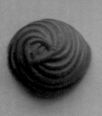

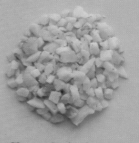

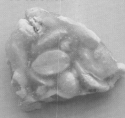

Chocolate hazelnut whirl
40 calories

Chopped mixed nuts
per 5ml (1 level teaspoon)
10 calories

Monkey nut
10 calories

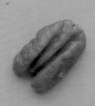

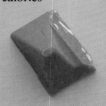

Almond
10 calories

Buttered Brazil
40 calories

Pecan nut (salted)
15 calories

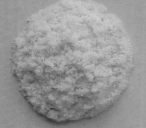

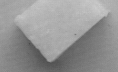

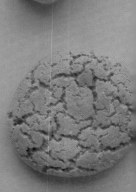

Pistachio nut
5 calories

Piece of coconut ice
110 calories

Macaroon
25 calories

Ground almonds
per 5ml (1 level teaspoon)
10 calories

The nut-eater's guide

Cashew nut (salted)
5 calories

Roasted salted peanut
5 calories

Crunchy nut topping
per 5ml (1 level teaspoon)
10 calories

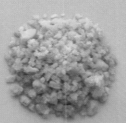

Chestnut
10 calories

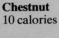
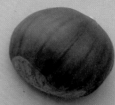

Desiccated coconut
per 5ml (1 level teaspoon)
10 calories

Chocolate Brazil
55 calories

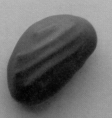

Piece of nut toffee
40 calories

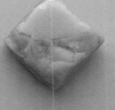

Macadamia nut
10 calories

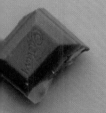

Square wholenut chocolate
10 calories

Hazelnut
5 calories

Coconut mushroom
25 calories

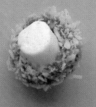

Chocolate almond
15 calories

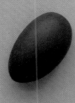

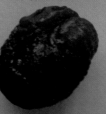

Marron glacé
45 calories

Maple Brazil
60 calories

Nutty Calorie Chart

Calories per 28g (1oz)

Almonds	160
Barcelona nuts	181
Brazil nuts	176
Cashew nuts	160
Chestnuts - shelled	48
Coconut - desiccated	171
Coconut - fresh	100
Hazelnuts	108
Monkeynuts	112
Peanut butter	177
Peanuts - roasted	162
Walnuts	149

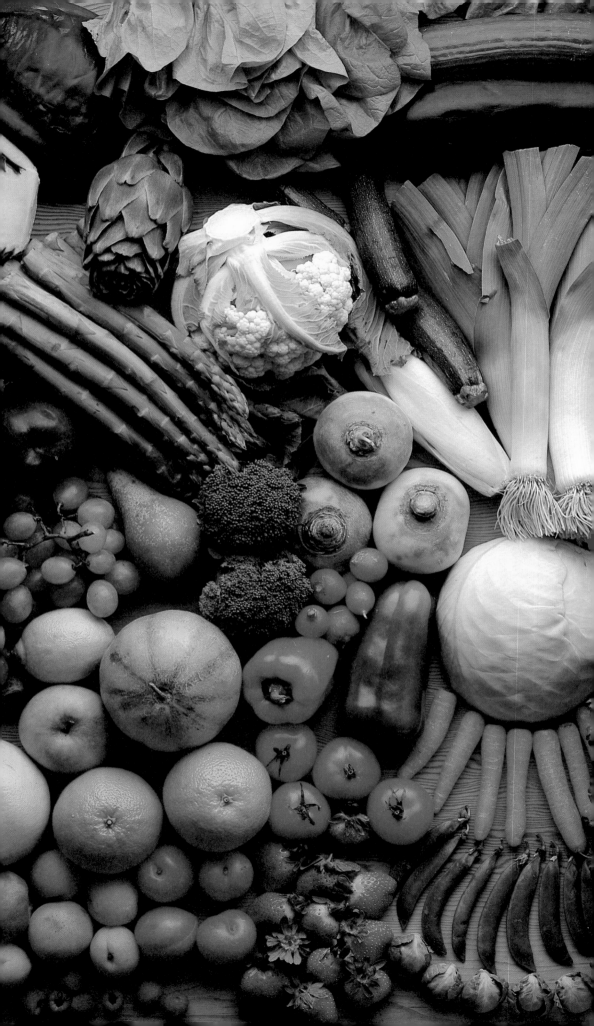

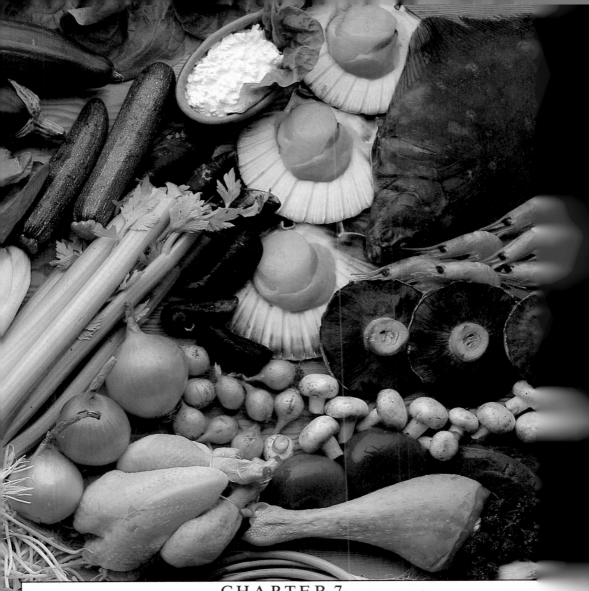

CHAPTER 7

Six diets to suit your lifestyle

All the diets in this chapter are guaranteed to see off excess weight at a fast rate, and there is one here that will work for you. The *Main Meal Diet* is tailor-made for anyone who can be super-strict during the day, but wants to sit down to a hearty meal in the evening. The *Metabolic Diet* allows you to eat five small meals a day and is ideal if you are a nibbler. The *Safety-Net Diet* is for anyone who feels they can't keep to a diet plan unless it allows some regular treats. If you don't eat meat, try the *Vegetarian Diet*. The *Superfoods Diet* is crammed full of all the foods which nutritionists recommend for maximum health and fitness and the *Speedy Packed Meal Diet* not only cuts down time in the kitchen, it can speed up your weight loss, too. Take a look at the diets in this chapter and choose the one that fits easily into your lifestyle. All of them allow you to choose exactly which meals you eat, but read on before you work out your weekly menus. A diet should not only help you to slim, it should make you feel fit and healthy, too.

All foods supply us with calories (simply another word for energy), and nearly all foods contain at least some of the nutrients that restore body tissue and are essential for the maintenance of good health. In modern Western society, few people go short of calories and many are overweight as a consequence of consuming far too many calories, which are stored by the body in the form of surplus fat.

Nutritional deficiencies are not prevalent in the West as, by eating generous amounts of a variety of foods, most people take in all the nutrients they need. However, when you are trying to eat less in order to shed weight, a little more care is needed to ensure that you get an adequate supply of vitamins, minerals and protein.

Nutritional requirements are usually stated in daily terms because these happen to be the most convenient and easily understood way of expressing them. In fact, the body can store most nutrients, although not all, and none is needed specifically on a daily basis. If you have been consuming food containing generous amounts of Vitamin A, for example, (found mainly in dairy products, liver and green vegetables), then it is unlikely that your body would run out of it if you didn't eat more for a very long time. On a Western-style diet, though, it would be difficult not to consume some Vitamin A. Water-soluble vitamins (such as Vitamin C) are stored by the body for a shorter period than the fat-soluble vitamins (such as Vitamin A), but as long as you eat a reasonably varied diet it is unlikely that you will ever go short.

How important is protein? If we eliminated protein from our diet completely, we would not survive for very long. Protein is the major component of all body cells and is being continually broken down and replaced. The minimum intake thought to guard the average person from protein deficiency has been reduced steadily over the years. As scientists' knowledge of the human body and its functioning increases, they can define its needs more accurately; but they feel it is safer to over-estimate what a body needs rather than set the recommended dose too low. The recommended intake of protein for an average woman in Britain is 54g (2oz) a day. You will usually get all you require from a variety of sources, such as milk, meat, fish, cereals, vegetables and bread.

Some misguided people seem to believe that a high-protein diet contains practically no calories but, like any other food substance, protein provides calories — in fact, as many as carbohydrates, compared weight for weight. You can grow as fat from eating an excess of high-protein foods as you can from consuming too much starch.

The easiest way to ensure that your diet contains all the essential nutrients is to choose one of the set diets included in this book. They have been designed to supply all you need for a healthy, and balanced diet. If you use the calorie charts at the back of the book to make up your own menus, follow the basic rule to vary meals each day, and include some fresh fruit, vegetables, lean meats, fish, cereals and low-fat dairy products. Green vegetables are useful to diets. One big plus is that, because their calorie counts are so low, you can afford to pile them on to your plate. And because you can eat them in large amounts, their nutritional contribution to your diet may be greater than you imagine. The prime factor in weighing up any food's worth is the quantity you are likely to eat. Liver perfectly illustrates this. Yes, it's one of the most nutritious foods you can consume — but are you likely to eat it more than a couple of times a week? Whereas green vegetables will probably make a daily appearance in your menus. The amount you serve will vary considerably, of course. Boiled Brussels sprouts weigh a lot, for example; you'd be unlikely to want a similar weight of lettuce leaves on your plate! Our chart shows average portions.

Although it is often said that vegetables lose their vitamins when cooked, in fact only Vitamin C and the B range of vitamins are at risk. There is no doubt that when you boil cabbage, or leave green vegetables soaking before cooking them, the Vitamin C content will seep out into the water. If you chop a lettuce and leave it standing for any length of time, Vitamin C tends to disappear, too.

But, when deciding if you will get more value from your vegetables raw or cooked, the real question you need to consider is how much are you likely to eat of each? Not all vegetables could be eaten raw, of course, but our research shows that you are likely to eat at least 175g (6oz) cooked cabbage, while you would probably eat less than half this amount if you served it raw in a coleslaw. The same goes for spinach, Brussels sprouts and peppers (capsicums). In all of these cases, even though cooking reduces Vitamin C, a cooked portion will give you more of that vitamin than the small weight you'd happily swallow raw. And because the Vitamin A and iron content doesn't change, you get lots more when you eat cooked vegetables.

Much more of your iron intake is likely to

come from meat, fish and beans, however, than from green vegetables. Choose low-fat meats — chicken or turkey eaten without their skin are obvious choices, but very lean beef or pork can also easily be incorporated into a slimming plan. Apart from its iron content, meat is also a good source of the B vitamins.

If you are a vegetarian, be sure to include some brown rice, lentils, beans or peas in your menus — all these foods are good for protein, fibre and other nutrients. Nutritional research now sets a daily intake of 30–40g of fibre as a good-health help. An average 115g (4oz) portion of boiled peas will give you 14g — almost half your daily minimum — and a 225g (7.9oz) can of baked beans in tomato sauce will give you 16g of fibre. The highest-fibre green-leaf vegetable is spinach. From an average 130g (4½oz) portion boiled spinach, you'd get 8g fibre. And, although weight-wise they don't rate as one of the highest-fibre green vegetables, Brussels sprouts are a good source (5g per average serving) because you'd probably eat a lot of them. Also worth a mention are broccoli, spring greens and runner beans. All green vegetables have a little fibre, but peppers (capsicums), lettuce and cucumber are unlikely to contribute very much to your daily total.

The following diets have been formulated to fit into a number of different life-styles, so the best one for you is the one that you can most easily keep to. Some slimmers will find that eating three regular meals a day provides their best dieting method. Others may discover that dieting is easier if they follow a completely different eating pattern. In fact, altering your meal times and adopting a less rigid, or different, pattern of eating can help to achieve long-term weight control.

Snack-eating urges can be enormously strong and hard to resist. If this is your main dieting downfall, try eating only when you really do experience a great eating urge. If you do not feel particularly hungry at breakfast time, skip that meal and save the calories for an emergency snack.

There is a widely-held belief that food eaten in the evening is more likely to turn into surplus fat than food that is eaten earlier in the day. This seems to have arisen from the notion that, if you do not exercise after eating, you do not burn up the calories and they are stored by the body as fat. The truth is that the body continues burning up calories even when you are asleep.

On the current evidence, it seems doubtful that any weight-losing advantages of eating earlier in the day are great enough to offset the late-evening willpower collapse that so often results in an illicit slice of cake or a TV snack. If you find that saving most of your calories for the evening is the surest way of keeping to your 1,000 or 1,500 calories target for the day, then we recommend that you continue dieting in this way.

When you follow one of the recommended diets, remember that there is no need to eat every single calorie each day. If you eat less food on an easy-to-diet day, you can 'bank' some of the left-over items of food for the next day, when your mood and circumstances may make it harder to keep to your allotted food allowance. Provided that your food intake averages out right, you will lose the same amount of weight.

The amount of weight you lose will depend on how accurately you stick to the diet, how overweight you are and for how long you have been dieting. Set yourself achievable weight-loss goals. Setting goals that are too large only leads to a feeling of despair when you inevitably fail. A reasonable weight loss would be 1kg (2lb) a week, although heavily overweight people often lose more than this, particularly in the first week. If you slip up and have an eating binge, remember that this does not signal the end of your diet. Undo any damage by switching to the *Speedy Packed Meal Diet* on page 126 for a few days, or follow one of the emergency day diets on page 170.

Read the introductions to your chosen diets, and follow the rules carefully. If you follow all the advice in this book as well as your eating plan, you *will* lose excess weight.

Green vegetables		Nutrients as % of recommended daily intake			
PER AVERAGE PORTION	CALS	VIT C	VIT A	IRON	FIBRE
50g (2oz) raw Brussels sprouts	15	170	5	3	8
175g (6oz) boiled Brussels sprouts	30	227	15	7	16
65g (2½oz) shredded raw white cabbage	16	76	trace	2	6
175g (6oz) boiled savoy cabbage	15	85	11	10	14
½ raw average pepper (capsicum)	11	237	3	2	2
150g (5oz) cooked pepper (capsicum)	20	284	6	5	4
50g (2oz) raw spinach	14	97	62	15	n/a
130g (4½oz) boiled spinach	41	107	170	43	27

n/a = figures not available

The main meal diet

This diet is tailor-made for anyone who is able to be super-strict during the day, but wants to sit down to a hearty meal in the evening. Dieting resolve is often at its strongest around breakfast time. But later on, weary from a hard day's work or from running around after the children, many a slimmer finds her willpower is at its lowest ebb. This is an excellent diet if you enjoy eating with the family in the evening, and dislike the idea of having to cook one meal for them and a separate dieting meal for yourself. It's also a good way to secretly slim an overweight husband — he'll probably never notice he's dieting!

You can select a main meal just for one, a main meal for two, or increase quantities to fit family numbers. The main meals are generous in quantity, but any non-dieting members of the family can add extra vegetables if they wish. If you have under 6kg (1st) to lose, here is what you do. During the day you select four items from the fruit list. You can either eat these a piece at a time, or chop the selection to make a fruit salad. If you make up a fruit salad, you can add a squeeze of lemon juice to prevent the fruit from turning brown. You are also allowed either 275ml (½ pint) skimmed milk to use in drinks — unsugared black coffee and tea is unlimited — or two small cartons of very

low-fat yogurt. This, together with your main meal, adds up to 1,000 calories a day.

If you have over 6kg (1st) to lose or if you are a man, you can increase your daily calories to 1,250 by selecting one item from the 250-calorie snack list. Men with over 6kg (1st) to lose and women with over 18kg (3st) to lose can eat an additional two items from the snacks list.

When you eat your daily main meal really doesn't matter. So if, say, you prefer at weekends to have your main meal at midday, then the diet will work perfectly well, as long as you keep to your daily calorie allowance.

The *Main Meal Diet* makes dieting simple for anyone who knows that her willpower waxes and wanes. For the comforting thought that a big plateful of nourishing food is not many hours away can really help to sustain your resolve.

Fruit list (50 calories per item)

Choose any four items each day
Apple, 1 medium
Apricots, dried, 5
Apricots, fresh, 200g (7oz)
Banana, 1 small
Cherries, fresh, 115g (4oz)
Currants, dried, 30ml
   (2 level tablespoons)
Dates, dried, 5, fresh, 3
Figs, dried, 2, fresh, 4
Gooseberries, ripe dessert,
   150g (5oz)
Grapefruit, 1 large
Grapes, 75g (3oz)
Kiwi fruit, 2 medium
Mango, ½ medium
Melon, 275g (10oz) weighed
   with skin
Nectarine, 1 medium
Orange, 1 medium
Peach, 1 large
Pear, 1 medium
Pineapple, 200g (7oz) slice
   weighed with skin
Plums, 3 medium
Prunes, 5
Raisins, 30ml (2 level
   tablespoons)
Raspberries, 200g (7oz)
Strawberries, 200g (7oz)
Sultanas, 30ml (2 level
   tablespoons)
Tangerines or Satsumas, 2 medium

Diet rules

1 Each day you may choose *one* main meal. You should vary these meals and, for good nutrition, try to have at least four different ones each week.
2 In addition to this meal, you may choose four portions from the fruit list. These may be eaten at any time of the day. They can be eaten separately or they can be chopped up and mixed together to make a fruit salad that you could dip into whenever you wish. A good squeeze of lemon juice may be added to a fruit salad to prevent it turning brown.
3 You may have 275ml (½ pint) skimmed milk each day to use in unsugared tea or coffee. If you do not use milk in your drinks, you may have 2 small cartons of very low-fat yogurt instead.
4 One main meal plus four pieces of fruit and your milk allowance adds up to 1,000 calories a day. If you have over 6kg (1st) to lose or are a man, you may also have a 250-calorie snack meal. Two additional snacks would bring your total up to 1,500 calories daily – a woman with over 18kg (3st) to lose and a man with over 6kg (1st) to go should still lose weight on this allowance.

Cod and Prawn Pie; Chicken Pilaf

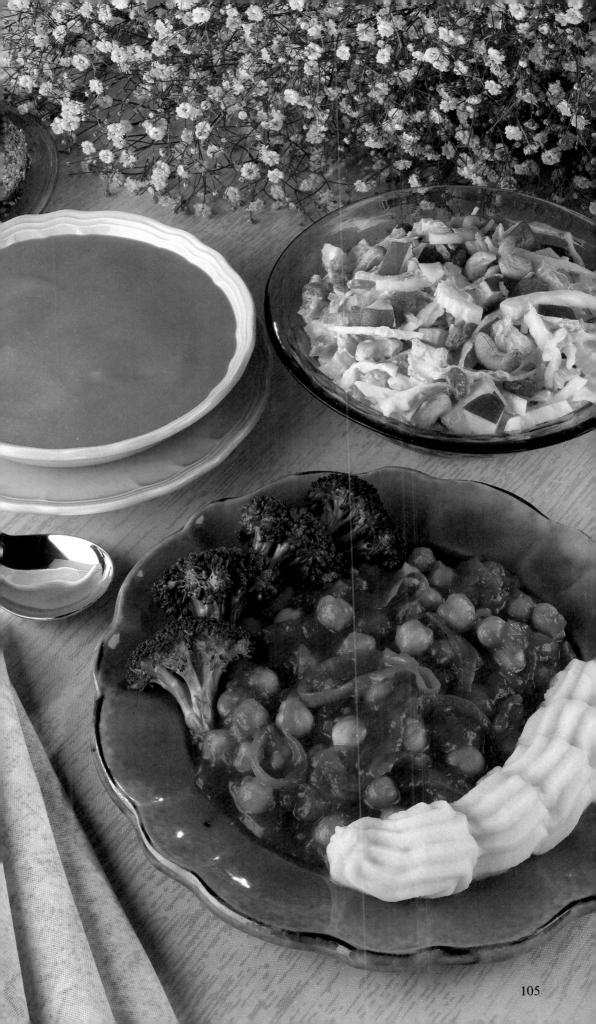

Toast and Jam or Marmalade

2 slices wholemeal bread (35g/1¼oz each)
10ml (2 level teaspoons) low-fat spread
10ml (2 level teaspoons) jam or marmalade

Toast the bread and top with low-fat spread and jam or marmalade.

Grapefruit, Boiled Egg and Bread

½ grapefruit
1 egg (size 3)
1 slice wholemeal bread (35g/1¼oz)
5ml (1 level teaspoon) low-fat spread

Eat the grapefruit. Boil the egg and serve with the bread and low-fat spread.

Light meals (300 calories)

Nutty Banana Sandwich; Biscuit

2 slices wholemeal bread (35g/1¼oz each)
5ml (1 level teaspoon) honey
2 walnut halves
1 small banana
1 small digestive or gingernut biscuit

Spread one slice of bread with honey. Roughly chop walnuts and mash banana. Make into a sandwich with bread. Follow with biscuit.

Salad Sandwich; Fruit

2 slices wholemeal bread (35g/1¼oz each)
15ml (1 level tablespoon) low-calorie
 mayonnaise
½ tomato
Few slices cucumber
Lettuce
Mustard and cress
1 medium banana or 150g (5oz) grapes

Spread the bread with mayonnaise. Make into a sandwich with the salad vegetables. Follow with the fruit.

Peanut Butter Sandwich; Fruit

2 slices wholemeal bread (35g/1¼oz each)
10ml (2 level teaspoons) peanut butter
1 medium banana or 1 large orange

Make sandwich with the bread and peanut butter. Follow with the fruit.

Cheese, Tomato and Pickle Sandwich

2 slices wholemeal bread (35g/1¼oz each)
5ml (1 level teaspoon) low-fat spread
15ml (1 level tablespoon) sweet pickle
1 small tomato
40g (1½oz) fat-reduced hard cheese

Spread one slice of bread with low-fat spread and one with pickle. Slice the tomato and make into a sandwich with the cheese.

Baked Beans on Toast; Fruit

227g (8oz) canned baked beans in tomato
 sauce
1 slice wholemeal bread (35g/1¼oz)
1 medium orange or small banana

Heat the baked beans. Toast the bread and serve the beans on top. Follow with the fruit.

Carrot and Potato Soup; Bread and Curd Cheese

175g (6oz) carrots
75g (3oz) potato
2.5ml (½ level teaspoon) ground coriander
2.5ml (½ level teaspoon) ground cumin
1 vegetable stock cube
275ml (½ pint) water
15g (½oz) powdered skimmed milk
Salt and pepper
1 slice wholemeal bread (35g/1¼oz)
15ml (1 level tablespoon) curd cheese

Slice the carrots and dice the potato. Place in a pan with the spices, stock cube and water. Bring to the boil, cover the pan and simmer gently for 20 minutes. Purée in a blender or food processor. Add the powdered skimmed milk and blend until evenly-mixed. Reheat and season to taste. Serve with the bread and curd cheese.

Butter Bean and Tomato Soup with Bread

½ small onion
227g (8oz) can butter beans
227g (8oz) canned tomatoes
¼ chicken or vegetable stock cube
115ml (4 fl oz) water
¼ bay leaf
2.5ml (½ level teaspoon) sugar
Dash Worcestershire sauce
1 slice wholemeal bread (35g/1¼oz)
5ml (1 level teaspoon) low-fat spread

Chop the onion and place in a saucepan with the butter beans and tomatoes (including the liquor from the cans). Add the stock cube, water, bay leaf, sugar and Worcestershire sauce. Bring to the boil, cover and simmer for 10 minutes. Discard the bay leaf. Purée the soup in a blender and then return to the pan to reheat. Serve with the bread and low-fat spread.

Crunchy Vegetable Salad

175g (6oz) cauliflower
2 spring onions
¼ red or green pepper (capsicum)
115g (4oz) canned sweetcorn
150g (5oz) canned or cooked red kidney
 beans
50g (2oz) bean sprouts
30ml (2 tablespoons) oil-free French
 dressing
Lettuce

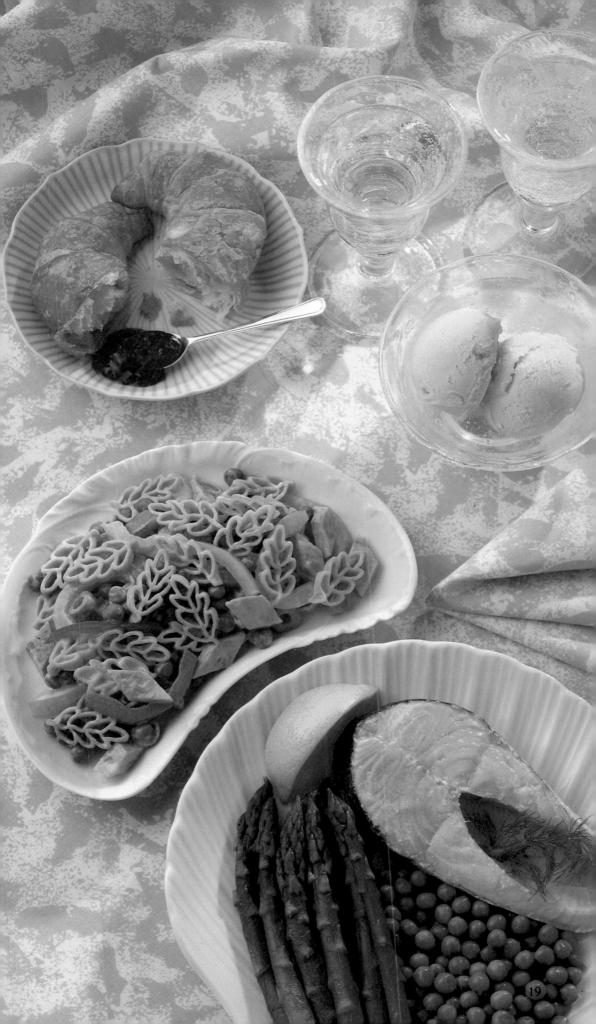

19

Toast with Banana and Honey

1 slice wholemeal bread (35g/1¼oz)
10ml (2 level teaspoons) honey
1 medium banana

Toast the bread and spread with honey. Mash the banana and place on top.

Cereal and Banana

25g (1oz) bran flakes or cornflakes or wheat flakes
1 small banana
150ml (¼ pint) skimmed milk

Slice the banana and mix with the cereal. Serve with the milk.

Cereal and Raisins

15ml (1 level tablespoon) raisins or sultanas
2 wheat breakfast biscuits
150ml (¼ pint) skimmed milk

Sprinkle the raisins or sultanas over the wheat biscuits. Serve with the milk.

Grapefruit; Scrambled Egg on Toast

½ grapefruit
1 egg (size 3)
15ml (1 tablespoon) skimmed milk
5ml (1 level teaspoon) low-fat spread
1 slice wholemeal bread (35g/1¼oz)

Eat the grapefruit. Lightly beat the egg and milk together. Place in a non-stick pan with the low-fat spread and cook gently, stirring. Toast the bread and serve the egg on top.

Lunches and evening meals
(300 calories)

Bacon Sandwich

70g (2½oz) back bacon
2 slices wholemeal bread (35g/1¼oz each)

Grill the bacon until well-cooked and make it into a sandwich with the bread.

Scrambled Egg and Smoked Salmon on Toast

25g (1oz) smoked salmon (end cuts are fine)
2 eggs (size 3)
15ml (1 tablespoon) skimmed milk
Pepper
5ml (1 level teaspoon) low-fat spread
1 slice wholemeal bread (35g/1¼oz)

Cut the smoked salmon into small pieces. Lightly beat the egg with the milk and season with pepper. Pour into a non-stick pan and add the low-fat spread. Cook over a low heat, stirring, until creamy. While it is cooking toast the bread. Stir the smoked salmon into the eggs and serve on the toast.

Chicken with Peas and Sweetcorn

175g (6oz) chicken breast with bone
115g (4oz) peas, frozen
115g (4oz) sweetcorn, frozen or canned

Grill the chicken until cooked through and then discard the skin. Boil the peas and frozen sweetcorn. Heat the sweetcorn.

Corned Beef and Pickle Sandwich

2 slices wholemeal bread (35g/1¼oz) each
15ml (1 level tablespoon) sweet pickle
5ml (1 level teaspoon) low-fat spread
50g (2oz) corned beef

Spread one slice of the bread with pickle and the other with low-fat spread. Make into a sandwich with the corned beef.

Chicken Roll and Chutney Sandwich; Fruit

2 slices wholemeal bread (35g/1¼oz) each
5ml (1 level teaspoon) low-fat spread
15ml (1 level tablespoon) mango chutney
25g (1oz) chicken roll or lean roast chicken
1 medium apple or pear

Spread one slice of bread with low-fat spread and one with chutney. Make into a sandwich with chicken. Follow with fruit.

Cauliflower Cheese

225g (8oz) cauliflower, fresh or frozen
15ml (1 level tablespoon) cornflour
150ml (¼ pint) skimmed milk
50g (2oz) fat-reduced hard cheese
Salt, pepper and mustard
15g (½oz) fresh wholemeal breadcrumbs

Boil the cauliflower until just tender. Drain thoroughly, place in a heatproof dish and keep warm. Mix the cornflour with a little milk until smooth. Add the remaining milk and pour into a saucepan. Bring to the boil, stirring continuously, and then simmer for a minute. Grate the cheese and add most to the sauce. Season with salt, pepper and a little mustard. Pour over the cauliflower. Sprinkle the remaining cheese and the breadcrumbs on top and grill until they brown.

Cheese and Ham Sandwich: Yogurt

25g (1oz) lean cooked ham
1 or 2 leaves lettuce
1 slice pumpernickel bread or wholemeal bread (40g/1½oz)
50g (2oz) cottage cheese with pineapple
½ peach, canned in fruit juice, drained
150g (5oz) natural low-fat yogurt

Discard all visible fat from the ham and then roll the slice up loosely. Place a little lettuce on bread and arrange ham at one end and the cottage cheese at the other end. Place peach in middle and serve. Follow with the yogurt.

Poached Salmon and Vegetables

200g (7oz) salmon steak
115g (4oz) asparagus, fresh, frozen or canned, drained
115g (4oz) peas, frozen
¼ lemon
Sprig dill, optional

Poach the salmon very gently in lightly-salted water for 10 minutes. Boil the asparagus and peas. Serve with the salmon, plus lemon, dill and vegetables.

Smoked Haddock with a Poached Egg and Bread

150g (5oz) smoked haddock fillet
1 egg (size 3)
1 slice wholemeal bread (35g/1¼oz)
7.5ml (1½ teaspoons) low-fat spread

Poach the smoked haddock in unsalted water until it flakes easily. Poach the egg in water or in a poacher greased with a little of the low-fat spread. Serve with the bread and remaining low-fat spread.

Pasta Salad

25g (1oz) wholewheat pasta shapes
50g (2oz) peas, frozen
50g (2oz) ham sausage
¼ red pepper (capsicum)
¼ yellow pepper (capsicum)
2 stuffed olives
30ml (2 level tablespoons) low-calorie salad cream

Boil the pasta until just tender. Boil the peas. Rinse both in cold water as soon as they are cooked and then drain them. Chop the ham sausage. Deseed the red and yellow pepper (capsicum) and cut into small strips. Slice olives. Mix ingredients together and serve.

Pastrami and Coleslaw with Rye Bread

75g (3oz) white cabbage
50g (2oz) carrot
2 spring onions
1 stick celery
15ml (1 level tablespoon) low-calorie salad cream
15ml (1 level tablespoon) natural low-fat yogurt
50g (2oz) pastrami
25g (1oz) light rye bread or 35g (1¼oz) wholemeal bread
10ml (2 level teaspoons) low-fat spread

Shred the cabbage and grate the carrot. Slice the spring onions and celery. Mix all the vegetables with the salad cream and yogurt and arrange on a plate with the pastrami. Spread the bread with low-fat spread and serve with the pastrami and coleslaw.

Bacon Omelet and Vegetables

115g (4oz) mushrooms
2 tomatoes
20g (¾oz) streaky bacon
2 eggs (size 3)
15ml (1 tablespoon) water
Salt and pepper
5ml (1 teaspoon) melted butter or oil

Boil the mushrooms. Grill the halved tomatoes and the bacon. Keep the vegetables warm and cut the bacon into small pieces. Lightly beat the eggs and water together and season. Brush the oil or butter over a small non-stick omelet pan and heat. Add the eggs and cook, lifting the edges and tilting the pan, until just set. Fill with the bacon and serve with the vegetables.

Pastrami and Coleslaw with Rye Bread

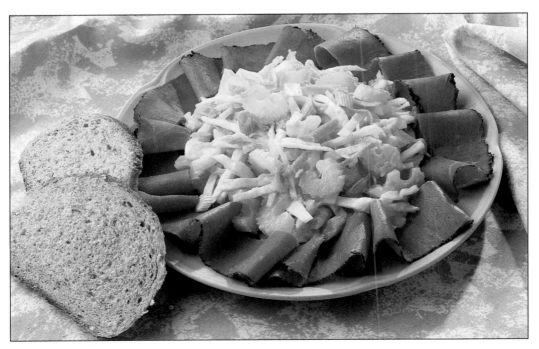

Chicken Drumsticks with Waldorf Salad

2 chicken drumsticks
2 sticks celery
15g (½oz) walnuts
1 medium apple
15ml (1 level tablespoon) low-calorie salad
cream
15ml (1 level tablespoon) natural low-fat
yogurt

Grill the drumsticks and then discard the skin. While they are cooking, slice the celery and roughly chop the walnuts. Core and dice the apple and mix with the celery, walnuts, salad cream and yogurt. Serve with the chicken.

Rollmop Herring and Beetroot and Apple Salad

75g (3oz) new potatoes
50g (2oz) boiled beetroot (not pickled)
2 sticks celery
25g (1oz) onion
1 small apple
30ml (2 level tablespoons) natural low-fat
yogurt
1 rollmop herring (70g/2½oz)

Scrub the potatoes and boil in their skins. Drain and cool. Cut potato and beetroot into small pieces. Slice celery. Thinly slice onion and divide into rings. Core and slice the apple. Mix all the ingredients except the herring together and serve with the fish.

Chicken Breast with Pepper Sauce

200g (7oz) chicken breast, part-boned
25g (1oz) onion
¼ clove garlic
115g (4oz) canned tomatoes, drained
weight
60ml (4 tablespoons) tomato juice from can
40g (1½oz) green pepper (capsicum)
40g (1½oz) red pepper (capsicum)
40g (1½oz) yellow pepper (capsicum)
Pinch mixed dried herbs
Salt and pepper
115g (4oz) whole green beans
115g (4oz) courgettes (zucchini)

Grill the chicken breast and then discard the skin. While it is cooking, make the sauce. Chop the onion and crush the garlic. Place in a pan with the tomatoes and their juice. Break up the tomatoes with a spoon. De-seed the peppers (capsicums) and cut into strips. Add these to the pan with the herbs and season. Bring to the boil, cover the pan and simmer gently for 15 minutes. Meanwhile, boil the beans and the courgettes (zucchini). Pour the peppers over the chicken and serve with the vegetables.

Kidney Risotto

25g (1oz) onion
25g (1oz) red pepper (capsicum)
40g (1½oz) long-grain brown rice
Pinch mixed dried herbs
5ml (1 level teaspoon) tomato purée
¼ beef stock cube
150ml (¼ pint) boiling water
115g (4oz) lamb's kidneys
50g (2oz) peas, frozen

Chop the onion and place in a small saucepan. Discard any white pith and seeds from the pepper (capsicum) and cut the flesh into small strips. Add to the pan with the rice, herbs and tomato purée. Dissolve the stock cube in the boiling water and add to the pan. Cover the pan, bring to the boil, and simmer for 10 minutes. Meanwhile, halve and core the kidneys and cut each half into two pieces. Add to the pan with the peas. Cover and simmer for another 20 minutes or until the rice is cooked. Check occasionally while rice is cooking. If the rice starts to stick, add a little extra boiling water.

Piperade

25g (1 oz) red pepper (capsicum)
25g (1oz) green pepper (capsicum)
1 tomato
1 spring onion
2 eggs (size 3)
15ml (1 tablespoon) skimmed milk
Salt and pepper
5ml (1 teaspoon) oil
1 slice wholemeal bread (35g/1¼oz)

Discard any white pith and seeds from the red and green pepper (capsicum). Chop the tomato and slice the spring onion. Lightly beat the eggs and milk together and season. Heat the oil in a small non-stick frying pan. Add the peppers and cook over a fairly low heat for 2–3 minutes. Add the tomato and spring onion and cook for another 2 minutes. Add the egg mixture and cook, stirring, until lightly-set. Serve with toast.

Tuna-stuffed Potato

200g (7oz) potato
50g (2oz) tuna in brine, drained
50g (2oz) cottage cheese with onion
5ml (1 level teaspoon) capers
Pepper

Scrub and prick the potato and bake in its jacket at 200°C, 400°F, gas mark 6, for about 1 hour or until soft when squeezed. Cut in half and scoop out the flesh. Mash with the tuna and cottage cheese. Chop the capers and stir in. Season with pepper. Pile back into the potato cases and reheat in the oven for 10 minutes.

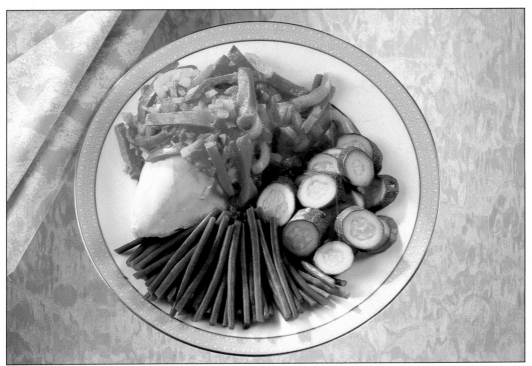

Chicken Breast with Pepper Sauce

Grilled Liver with Peppers and Runner Beans

½ green pepper (capsicum)
½ red pepper (capsicum)
½ small onion
½ clove garlic, optional
115g (4oz) canned tomatoes, drained
60ml (4 tablespoons) tomato juice from can
2.5ml (½ level teaspoon) sugar
Pinch dried mixed herbs
75g (3oz) runner beans or frozen sliced
  green beans
115g (4oz) lamb's liver
2.5ml (½ teaspoon) oil

Deseed the red and green pepper (capsicum) and cut the flesh into strips. Place in a small saucepan. Chop the onion and crush the garlic. Add to the pan with the tomatoes, juice, sugar and herbs. Break the tomatoes up roughly with a spoon and stir to mix. Cover the pan, bring to the boil and simmer gently for 15–20 minutes. Boil the runner beans. Brush the liver with oil and grill until just cooked. Serve with the peppers and runner beans.

Kidneys, Bacon and Baked Beans

2 lamb's kidneys
1 tomato
35g (1¼oz) back bacon
150g (5oz) canned baked beans in tomato
  sauce

Halve and core the kidneys. Halve the tomato. Grill the kidney and tomato lightly and grill the bacon until crisp. Heat the baked beans. Serve.

Ham Steak with Pineapple

1 bacon or ham steak (115g/4oz)
115g (4oz) broad beans
115g (4oz) carrots
1 ring pineapple canned in fruit juice,
  drained

Grill the ham or bacon steak. Boil the broad beans and carrots. Heat the pineapple under the grill and serve with the meat and vegetables.

Kidney Curry and Rice

25g (1oz) long-grain brown rice
25g (1oz) onion
5ml (1 teaspoon) oil
2.5ml (½ level teaspoon) curry powder
115ml (4 fl oz) water
15 ml (1 level tablespoon) mango chutney
10 ml (2 level teaspoons) tomato purée
115g (4oz) lamb's kidneys
5ml (1 level teaspoon) cornflour

Boil the rice. While it is cooking, make the sauce. Chop the onion and place in a small saucepan with the oil. Cook until soft. Stir in the curry powder and cook for 1–2 minutes. Add the water, mango chutney and tomato purée. Halve and core the kidneys and then cut each half into two pieces. Add to the pan. Cover, bring to the boil and simmer for 15 minutes. Mix the cornflour with a little cold water and stir into the kidneys. Bring to the boil, stirring continuously, and simmer for a minute. Drain the rice and serve with the curry.

Safety-net swaps (100 calories)

Sultanas or Raisins
40g (1½oz) sultanas or raisins

Dates
10 dried dates

Figs
3 dried figs

Peppermints
25g (1oz) peppermints

Fruit Pastilles
40g (1½oz) fruit pastilles

Liquorice Allsorts
35g (1¼oz) liquorice allsorts

Toasted Crumpet or Muffin
1 crumpet or muffin
5ml (1 level teaspoon) low-fat spread
5ml (1 level teaspoon) honey or jam

Toast the crumpet and top with the honey or jam.

Chocolate Finger Biscuits
4 chocolate finger biscuits

Chocolate Nut Cookies
2 medium-sized chocolate nut cookies

Ginger Nuts
2 medium ginger nut biscuits

Ice-cream
50g (2oz) ice-cream, vanilla or raspberry ripple or strawberry

Sorbet
75g (3oz) sorbet or water ice, any flavour

Fruit and Yogurt Meringue Nest
1 meringue nest
50g (2oz) raspberries or strawberries
45ml (3 level tablespoons) very low-fat fruit yogurt

Hull and slice the strawberries, if used. Mix the fruit with the yogurt and pile into the meringue nest.

Safety-net swaps (200 calories)

Chocolate Digestives
3 medium-sized chocolate digestive biscuits or graham crackers

Rich Tea Biscuits
5 round rich tea biscuits

Custard Creams
3 custard cream biscuits

Jam Doughnut
1 jam doughnut (70g/2¾oz)

Currant Bun and Butter
1 currant bun (45g/1¾oz)
7g (¼oz) butter

Split the currant bun and spread with butter.

Buttered Toasted Teacake
1 teacake (50g/2oz)
7g (¼oz) butter

Split and toast the teacake. Spread with butter.

Chips
130g (4½oz) grill chips or oven chips
Salt, optional
Vinegar, optional

Cook the chips as instructed on the packet and serve with salt and vinegar if liked.

Crisps and Fruit
1 packet potato crisps, (30g/1⅛oz), any flavour
1 medium pear or apple

Wine
2 glasses dry or medium red or white wine (150ml/5 fl oz each)

Beer or Cider or Lager
575ml (1 pint) beer or lager or medium sweet cider

Sherry
3 small schooners of sherry, any type (50ml/⅓ gill each)

Pineapple Alaska
1 egg white (size 3)
25g (1oz) caster sugar
1 ring pineapple canned in fruit juice, drained
40g (1½oz) vanilla ice-cream
¼ glacé cherry, optional
2 leaves angelica, optional

Preheat the oven to 220°C, 425°F, gas mark 7. Whisk the egg white until stiff. Add half the sugar and whisk until really stiff again. Fold in the remaining sugar. Place the pineapple on an ovenproof dish and top with the ice-cream. Cover with the meringue and bake in the oven for 2–4 minutes or until the edges of the meringue start to brown. Decorate with cherry and angelica, if liked, and serve immediately.

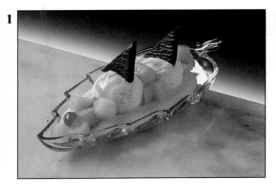
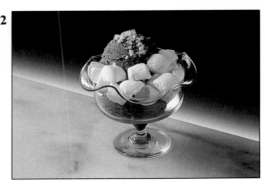

1 *Banana Split;* **2** *Rocky Road Sundae*

Banana and Custard

15ml (1 level tablespoon) custard powder
10ml (2 level teaspoons) sugar
150ml (¼ pint) skimmed milk
1 medium banana

Mix the custard powder and sugar with a little milk until smooth. Add the rest of the milk and pour into a small pan. Bring to the boil, stirring all the time and simmer for 1–2 minutes. Slice the banana into a bowl and pour the custard on top.

Rice Pudding

227g (8oz) canned rice pudding

Serve the rice pudding hot or cold.

Safety-net swaps (300 calories)

Chocolate Mousse

25g (1oz) plain chocolate
1 egg (size 3)
10ml (2 teaspoons) brandy or black coffee
15ml (1 tablespoon) double cream

Melt the chocolate in a shallow bowl over a pan of hot, not boiling, water. Make sure no water or steam comes in contact with the chocolate. Remove from the heat. Separate the egg and add the yolk to the chocolate, stirring briskly. Add the brandy or coffee. Whisk the white until stiff and fold in gently. Turn the Chocolate Mousse into a dish and chill until set. Spoon the cream over the surface and serve.

Banana Split

1 small banana
75g (3oz) vanilla ice cream
75g (3oz) fruit cocktail canned in fruit juice, drained
15ml (1 level tablespoon) raspberry or strawberry ice-cream topping
1 chocolate mint

Cut the banana in half lengthways and place on a shallow dish. Arrange the ice-cream in the middle and top with the fruit cocktail. Spoon the sauce over the fruit. Cut the chocolate mint in half and use to decorate the Banana Split.

Rocky Road Sundae

40g (1½oz) marshmallows
75g (3oz) chocolate ice-cream
5ml (1 level teaspoon) chopped nuts

Roughly chop the marshmallows. Place the ice-cream in a dish and surround with the marshmallows. Sprinkle the nuts on top.

French Bread and Cheese

50g (2oz) French bread
40g (1½oz) Philadelphia or Fetta cheese

Spread French bread with cheese.

Cheese and Biscuits

*50g (2oz) Brie or Camembert or Roquefort cheese **or** 40g (1½oz) Cheddar cheese*
4 water biscuits
2 sticks celery

Serve cheese on biscuits and eat with celery.

Toffee

70g (2½oz) toffees or caramels

Boiled Sweets

90g (3¼oz) boiled sweets

Croissant and Jam

1 croissant (65g/2½oz)
10ml (2 level teaspoons) jam

Serve the croissant with the jam.

Nuts

50g (2oz) packet roasted salted or dry roasted cashew nuts or peanuts

Chocolate Eclair

75g (3oz) chocolate eclair with fresh cream

Fruit Cake

50g (2oz) rich fruit cake, with or without icing and marzipan

Chocolate Cake

65g (2¼oz) chocolate cake with chocolate icing and butter icing filling

Chocolate

50g (2oz) bar chocolate, milk or plain

The speedy packed meal diet

If you've been slimming for some time and find your weight loss is slowing down, or if you want an emergency diet to rid you of a little excess weight in time for a special event, this diet is ideal. Your daily calorie total will be just 900 and that's low enough to lose weight at a speedy rate. The *Speedy Packed Meal Diet* is simple to follow, too. It takes just a few minutes each day to prepare and it's totally portable. It will steer you clear of the kitchen and its temptations, and free you to get out and about or to take extra exercise (strongly recommended if you want to lose weight quickly). Remember, though, that you should not eat for about two hours before any strenuous activity, such as swimming, doing a dance class or jogging. So exercise first and eat later – you'll find it more enjoyable that way, too.

Each day you choose one simple breakfast. After breakfast – it's always best to prepare food when you've just eaten, as there is less chance of indulging in snacking then – you prepare your other meals for the day. You are allowed one Packed Meal a day, but how you eat it is entirely up to you. You may divide it into two same-size meals if you wish, or you can eat a little for lunch and leave a larger portion for your main meal in the evening. If you are a nibbler by nature, you may well prefer to divide your day's food into four mini-meals. Just do what makes dieting easiest for you. Remember,

---

Diet rules

1 Each day, choose *one* breakfast from the list that follows. You can have the same one each day, or vary them if you wish. If you do not normally eat breakfast, save this meal to eat as a snack later in the day.
2 Each day choose *one* Packed Meal from the list that follows. You can select your favourites, but for good nutrition you should have at least four different Packed Meals each week.
3 You are allowed 275ml (½ pint) skimmed milk to use in drinks. Milk used in a breakfast or a Packed Meal is extra to this allowance. You may also drink unlimited black coffee and tea (unsugared), water, low-calorie squashes and low-calorie carbonated drinks.
4 One breakfast, one Packed Meal and 275ml (½ pint) milk amounts to 900 calories. This is a strict diet for a fast weight loss. After two weeks, if you still have weight to lose, you should add an extra 100 calories a day to bring your total up to 1,000 calories – the lowest number you should slim on for a longer-term plan.

---

though, if you have eaten everything by midday, you will have to wait until breakfast the next day before you eat again!

All the Packed Meals can be eaten cold, so you could pack up a picnic and have a completely portable dieting away-day. These meals are also very convenient if you need to take lunch to work.

Some of the Packed Meals can be eaten hot, so choose one of these if you prefer something warming in the evening. This diet is simple, effective and fun. Start today to send that surplus weight packing!

Breakfasts

Bran Cereal
40g (1½oz) bran breakfast cereal
150ml (¼ pint) skimmed milk

Serve the cereal with the milk.

Porridge
25g (1oz) instant oat cereal
150ml (¼ pint) skimmed milk

Heat the milk and mix with the cereal. Serve hot.

Puffed Wheat and Banana
1 small banana
15g (½oz) Puffed Wheat
150ml (¼ pint) skimmed milk

Slice the banana and mix with the cereal. Serve with the milk.

Toast and Marmalade with Juice
1 slice wholemeal bread (35g/1¼oz)
5ml (1 level teaspoon) low-fat spread
10ml (2 level teaspoons) jam or marmalade
115ml (4 fl oz) unsweetened grapefruit juice

Toast the bread and spread with low-fat spread and jam or marmalade. Drink juice.

Boiled Egg and Crispbreads
1 egg (size 3)
2 crispbreads
10ml (2 level teaspoons) low-fat spread

Boil egg. Serve with crispbreads and spread.

Yogurt with Orange
150g (5oz) natural low-fat yogurt
1 medium orange

Serve yogurt with segmented orange.

Leek and Potato Soup; Fruit and Yogurt;
Rice and Prawn Salad; Carrot and Bean Salad

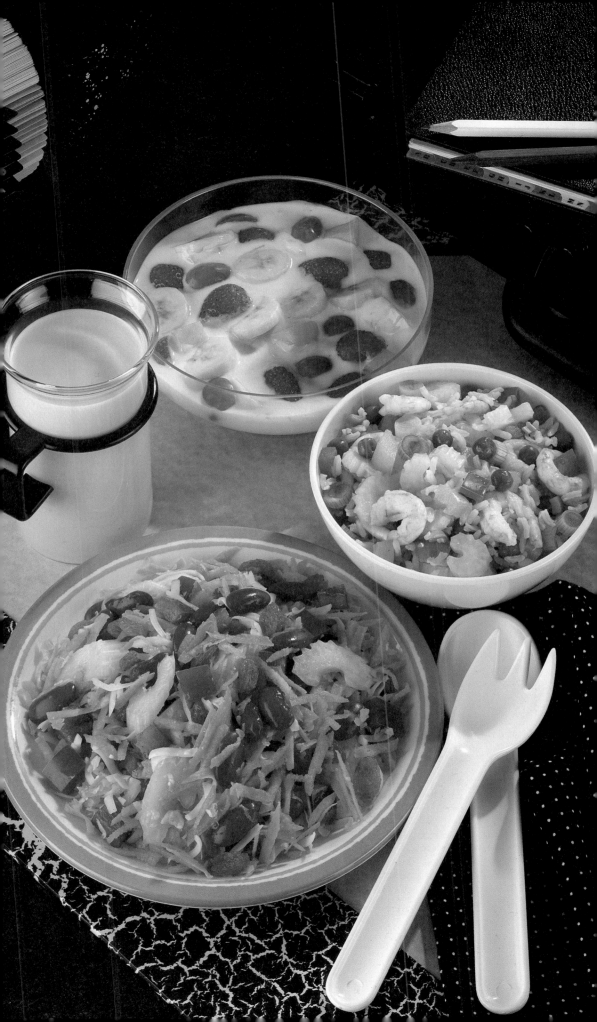

Packed meals

Pea and Bacon Soup

1 medium onion
1 stick celery
115g (4oz) potatoes, peeled weight
450g (1lb) frozen peas
1 chicken stock cube
5ml (1 level teaspoon) mixed dried
    herbs
850ml (1½ pints) water
115g (4oz) lean raw gammon rasher
15g (½oz) powdered skimmed milk
Salt and pepper
8 bread sticks

Slice the onion, potato and celery. Place in
a large pan with the frozen peas, stock cube,
herbs and water. Discard all visible fat from
the gammon or bacon and add to the pan.
Bring to the boil, cover the pan and simmer
for 30 minutes. Remove the gammon or
bacon and cut into small pieces. Purée the
soup in a blender or food processor until
smooth. Add the powdered milk and blend
until smooth again. Stir in the gammon or
bacon. Can be served hot or cold. If to be
eaten hot, reheat one portion and pour into
a vacuum flask. Keep the remainder in the
refrigerator and reheat when needed. If to
be served cold, allow to cool, then divide
into portions and refrigerate.

Pumpkin Soup

900g (2lbs) pumpkin; weighed without skin
175g (6oz) potatoes, peeled weight
50g (2oz) carrots, peeled weight
1 medium onion
2 chicken or vegetable stock cubes
1.15 litres (2 pints) water
Pinch allspice
Salt and pepper
25g (1oz) skimmed milk powder
75g (3oz) wholemeal bread

Cut the pumpkin and the potatoes into small
cubes. Slice the carrot and the onion. Place
all the vegetables in a saucepan with the
stock cubes, water and allspice. Cover the
pan, bring it to the boil, and simmer for 30
minutes. Purée the mixture in a blender or
food processor. Add the milk powder and
blend it in well. Season to taste with salt and
pepper. Cool and refrigerate until needed.
Toast the bread and leave it to cool. Cut it
into small cubes and keep them in a covered
container. Reheat a portion of the soup
when needed and sprinkle a few toast
croûtons on top before serving. For a packed
lunch, reheat the soup and carry it in a
vacuum flask. Pack the croûtons in a separate container.

Vegetable Broth

150g (5oz) potatoes, peeled weight
115g (4oz) parsnips, peeled weight
175g (6oz) swedes, peeled weight
115g (4oz) carrots, peeled weight
175g (6oz) leeks, white part only
1 medium onion
3 chicken or vegetable stock cubes
1.7 litres (3 pints) water
2 bay leaves
5ml (1 level teaspoon) mixed herbs
50g (2 oz) medium oatmeal
Salt and pepper

Cut the potato, parsnips, swedes and carrots
into small cubes. Chop the leeks and onion.
Place all the vegetables in a large pan with
the stock cubes, water, bay leaves, herbs and
oatmeal. Season with salt and pepper. Cover
the pan and bring to the boil, stirring frequently. Simmer for 1 hour, stirring occasionally. Pour one portion into a vacuum
flask, if necessary. Leave the rest to cool and
then refrigerate. Reheat a portion at a time
when needed.

Aduki Bean and Mushroom Salad

115g (4oz) aduki beans
115g (4oz) button mushrooms
4 spring onions
4 sticks celery
1 red pepper (capsicum)
115g (4 oz) ham sausage
60ml (4 tablespoons) oil-free French
    dressing
Salt and pepper

Soak the aduki beans overnight. Drain and
then boil them in fresh water until they are
tender (about 45 minutes). Drain them again
and leave to cool. Slice the mushrooms,
spring onions and celery. Discard the seeds
and white pith from the red pepper (capsicum) and dice the flesh. Dice the ham
sausage. Mix all the ingredients together,
add the French dressing and season lightly
with salt and pepper. Keep in the refrigerator
until needed.

Beef and Piccalilli French Bread

150g (5oz) French bread
75g (3oz) piccalilli
115g (4oz) lean roast topside of beef
Cucumber
Lettuce
Chicory
Mustard and cress

Cut the bread into two pieces. Halve and
spread with piccalilli. Discard all visible fat
from the beef and make onto two sandwiches with the bread and any of the salad
vegetables listed above.

Leek and Potato Soup

225g (8oz) leeks, white part only
1 stick celery
225g (8oz) potatoes, peeled weight
700ml (1¼ pints) water
2 chicken stock cubes
115 g (4oz) fromage frais (8 per cent fat)
Salt and pepper
75g (3oz) wholemeal bread

Slice the leeks, celery and potatoes and place in a saucepan with the water and stock cubes. Cover the pan, bring to the boil and simmer gently for 40 minutes or until the vegetables are tender. Purée until smooth. Add the cheese and season to taste. Can be served hot or cold. For hot soup, reheat one portion in a saucepan, then keep in a vacuum flask. Cool and refrigerate the remainder and reheat as needed. For chilled soup, divide into two portions, cool and refrigerate. Serve with wholemeal bread – toasted if you wish.

Chicken and Apricot Sandwiches

115g (4oz) cooked chicken, no skin
½ green or red pepper (capsicum)
4 ready-to-eat dried apricots
15ml (1 level tablespoon) low-calorie salad cream
15ml (1 level tablespoon) natural low-fat yogurt
15ml (1 level tablespoon) apricot chutney
6 small slices wholemeal bread (25g/1oz each)

Chop the chicken, pepper (capsicum) and apricots. Mix with the salad cream, yogurt and chutney. Divide the filling between three slices of bread and make into sandwiches with the remaining slices. Divide into portions, then wrap and refrigerate.

Humus and Crispbreads

175g (6oz) canned or cooked chick peas
60ml (4 tablespoons) liquid from can or cooking liquid
½ clove garlic
30ml (2 level tablespoons) tahini (sesame seed paste)
75g (3oz) cottage cheese with chives
Salt and paprika
3 sticks celery
5 crispbreads

Place the chick peas in a blender with the liquid, crushed garlic, tahini and cottage cheese. Purée until smooth. Add a little extra cooking liquid or liquid from the can if necessary to give the consistency of a thick dip. Season to taste with a little salt. Divide into two portions and refrigerate. Wash the celery and cut into short lengths. Divide into portions and refrigerate. Eat the humus with the celery sticks and crispbreads.

Carrot and Bean Salad

275g (10oz) carrots
50g (2oz) Edam cheese
2 green peppers (capsicums)
4 sticks celery
50g (2oz) raisins or sultanas
225g (8oz) red kidney beans, canned or cooked

Grate the carrot and the cheese. Dice the peppers and slice the celery. Mix all the ingredients together. Keep in the refrigerator in covered containers.

Pasta, Pepper and Chicken Salad

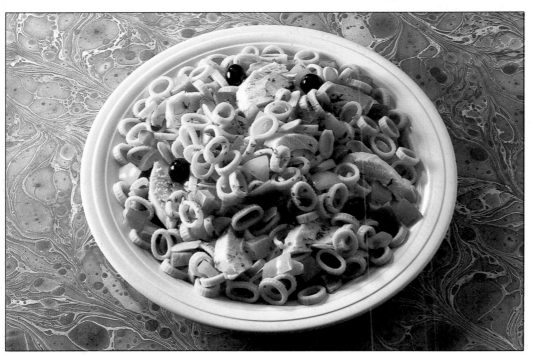

Seafood Ratatouille

450g (1lb) aubergines
450g (1lb) courgettes (zucchini)
1 red pepper (capsicums)
1 green pepper (capsicum)
2 onions
225g (8oz) French beans or whole green
  beans
2 × 400g (14oz) canned tomatoes.
2 cloves garlic
10ml (2 level teaspoons) dried oregano
10ml (2 level teaspoons) dried basil
150g (5oz) peeled prawns
150g (5oz) cooked mussels
Salt and pepper

Cut the aubergines into small cubes and slice the courgettes (zucchini). Sprinkle with salt and leave to stand for 20 minutes. Slice the red and green peppers (capsicums) and onions. Rinse the salt from the aubergines and courgettes (zucchini) and place them in a saucepan with peppers (capsicums), onions, beans and tomatoes and their juice. Crush garlic and add to pan with oregano and basil. Bring vegetables to the boil, cover and cook for 15 minutes. Add a little water towards the end of cooking if necessary to prevent the mixture sticking to the pan. Leave to cool. Stir in prawns and mussels. Cover and refrigerate. Serve hot or cold. If served hot only reheat one portion of the Seafood Ratatouille at a time.

Potato and Bacon Salad

2 eggs (size 3)
275g (10oz) potatoes (preferably small new
  ones)
115g (4oz) frozen peas
50g (2oz) streaky bacon
½ medium onion
½ red or green pepper (capsicum)
½ clove garlic, optional
45ml (3 tablespoons) unsweetened apple
  juice
15ml (1 tablespoon) white wine vinegar or
  cider vinegar
1 pickled walnut
Endive, watercress or shredded lettuce

Hard-boil the eggs. Scrub the potatoes and boil in their skins until almost tender. Add the peas and boil for 5 minutes or until potatoes are cooked through. Drain and cool. If the potatoes are large, cut them into cubes. Grill the bacon until crisp. Break into small pieces. Slice the onion and dice the pepper (capsicum). Crush the garlic if used and mix with the apple juice and wine vinegar. Chop the pickled walnut. Shell and slice the eggs and mix with the potatoes, peas, bacon, onion, pepper, dressing and pickled walnut. Divide into portions and keep in the refrigerator. Serve each portion on a little endive or watercress or shredded lettuce.

Pasta, Pepper and Chicken Salad

115g (4oz) wholewheat pasta shapes or
  macaroni
½ yellow pepper (capsicum)
1 green or red pepper (capsicum)
115g (4oz) cooked chicken, no skin
15ml (1 level tablespoon) toasted flaked
  almonds
5 black olives
60ml (4 tablespoons) oil-free French
  dressing
Chopped parsley, optional

Boil the pasta in lightly-salted water. Drain, rinse in cold water and drain again. Dice pepper (capsicum). Cut chicken into small bite-sized pieces. Mix the pasta, peppers and chicken with the almonds, olives and dressing. Sprinkle with a little parsley if liked. Divide into portions and keep in the refrigerator.

Rice and Prawn Salad

100g (3½oz) long-grain brown rice
115g (4oz) frozen peas
4 sticks celery
3 spring onions
1 red or green pepper (capsicum)
1 yellow pepper (capsicum)
225g (8oz) cucumber
115g (4oz) peeled prawns
45ml (3 tablespoons) oil-free French
  dressing

Boil the rice until tender. Boil the peas for 5 minutes. Drain rice and peas, rinse in cold water and drain again. Slice the celery and spring onions. Dice the pepper (capsicum) and cucumber. Mixll the ingredients together. Divide into portions and refrigerate.

Strawberry Cheese and Crispbreads

225g (8oz) strawberries
450g (1lb) cottage cheese with pineapple
7 crispbreads

Hull and slice the strawberries and mix with the cottage cheese. Divide into portions and refrigerate. Eat with crispbreads.

Fruit and Yogurt

150g (5oz) carton natural low-fat yogurt
2 × 150g (5oz) cartons very-low-fat fruit
  yogurt
1 large banana
1 medium mango
225g (8oz) strawberries
225g (8oz) seedless grapes

Mix the yogurts together in a large bowl. Peel and slice the banana and add to the yogurt. Peel, stone and cube the mango, then hull the strawberries. Add to the yogurt with grapes and mix gently. Divide into portions and keep covered in refrigerator.

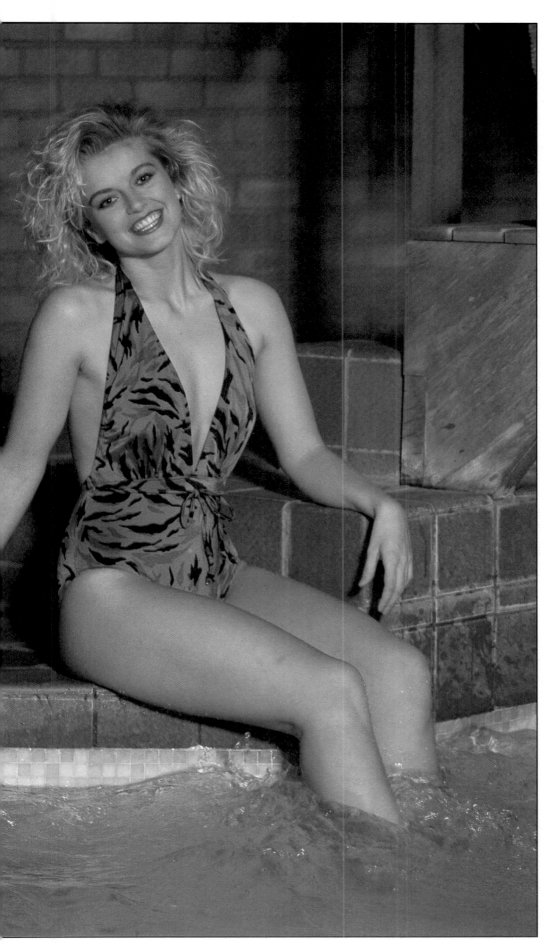

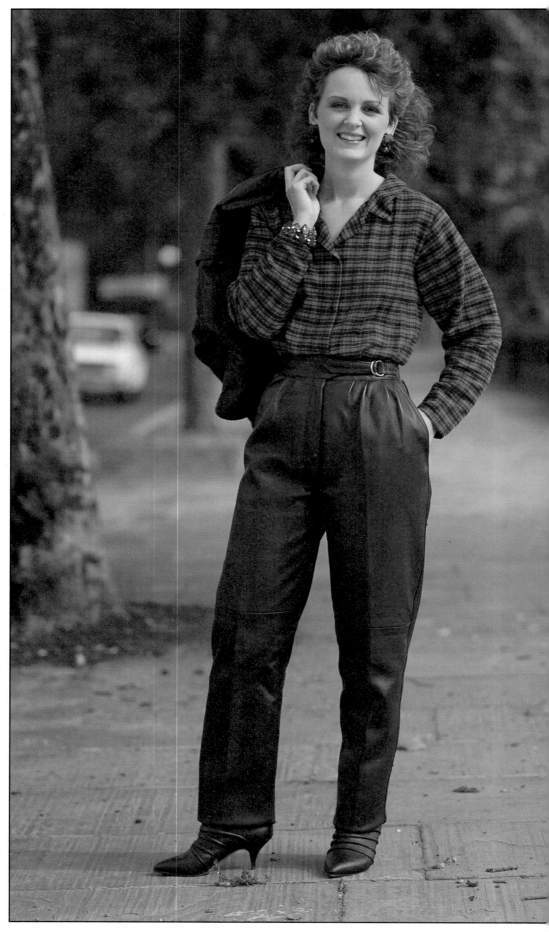

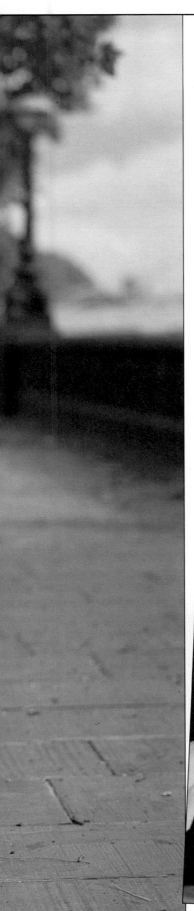

The 'other woman' was Sally

If any one had told Sally Mason that she would one day need to lose weight, she would have laughed. When she married Chris at 19, she was 1.65m (5ft 5in), took size-12 in clothes and weighed just 57.3kg (9st). But, by the time Ryan was born a couple of years later, her weight had shot up to 89kg (14st). And just before the arrival of James, her second baby, the scales actually hovered round the 100kg (16st) mark. Sally knew she had to slim. She built up dieting menus with the help of *Slimming Magazine*. As the weight began to disappear — at a steady 1–1.5kg (2–3lb) a week — Sally decided she wanted to be fit as well as un-fat. Some of her girlfriends used to go along to the Ladies' Night at the local baths, so she decided to join them. At first, it was a matter of just doing a couple of laboured widths across the pool, but then she built up to 10 lengths and a couple of weeks later could do 15. Eventually, she was swimming 30 lengths at each session.

Sally had less than 6kg (1st) to go when losing weight seemed to get harder. So she looked for an incentive to spur her on. Out of the blue came the chance to take part in a sponsored slim. She needed to lose 3.6kg (8lb) in four weeks. On the final day, she stepped on the scales and saw them register exactly 57.7kg (9st 1lb). She'd reached her target and raised money for charity. She had lost 30kg (5st) in nine months and at last was able to buy the really trim-fitting trousers and jeans she had always longed to wear. A little while after she had reached target, John, an old colleague of her husband's, called at their home. As all her attempts at airy chat seemed to fall on barren ground, Sally later asked her husband what had been the matter with John. It appeared that he had thought Sally had left home and Chris had got himself a new young woman . . . well, in a way, he had!

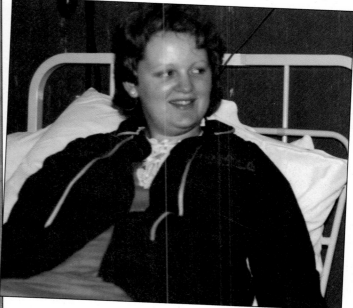

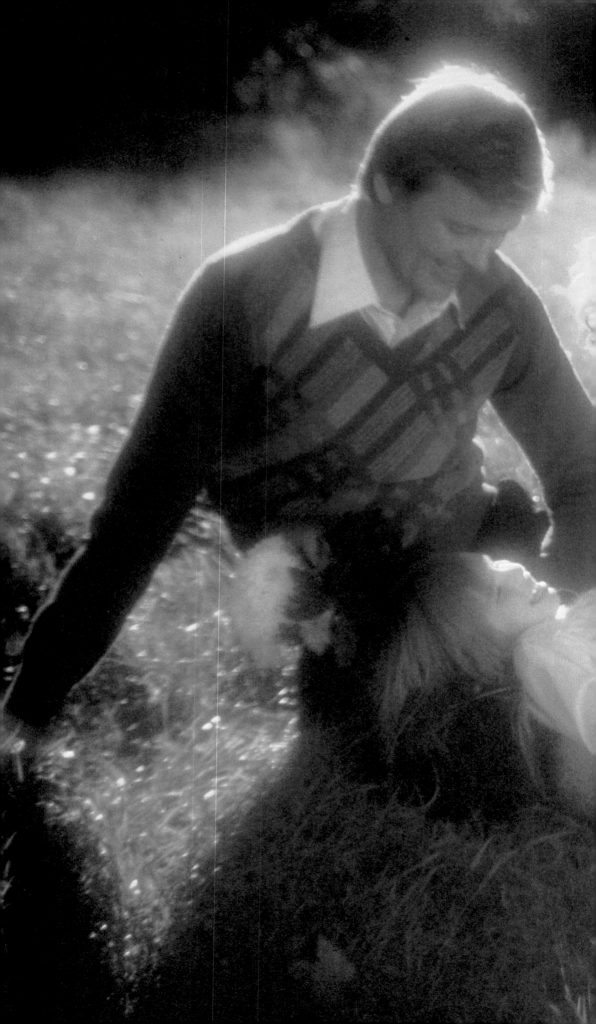

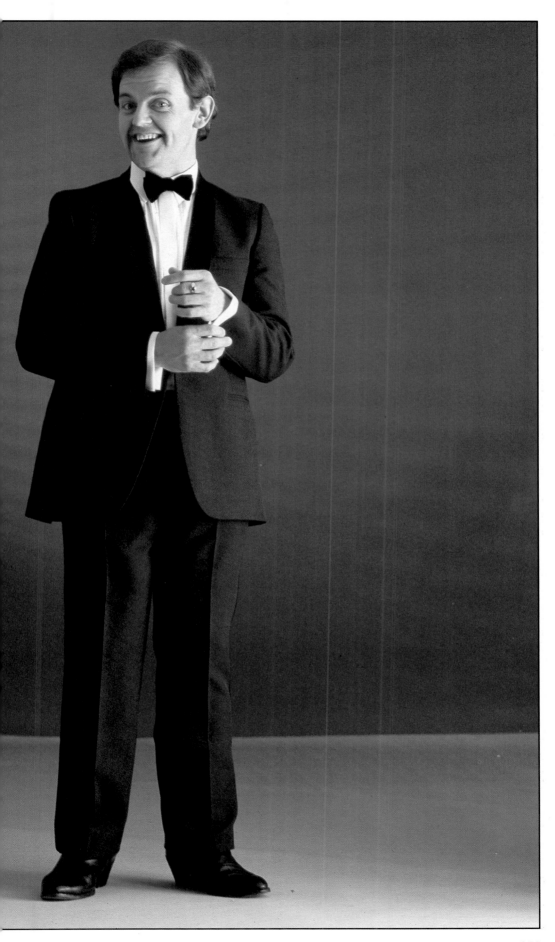

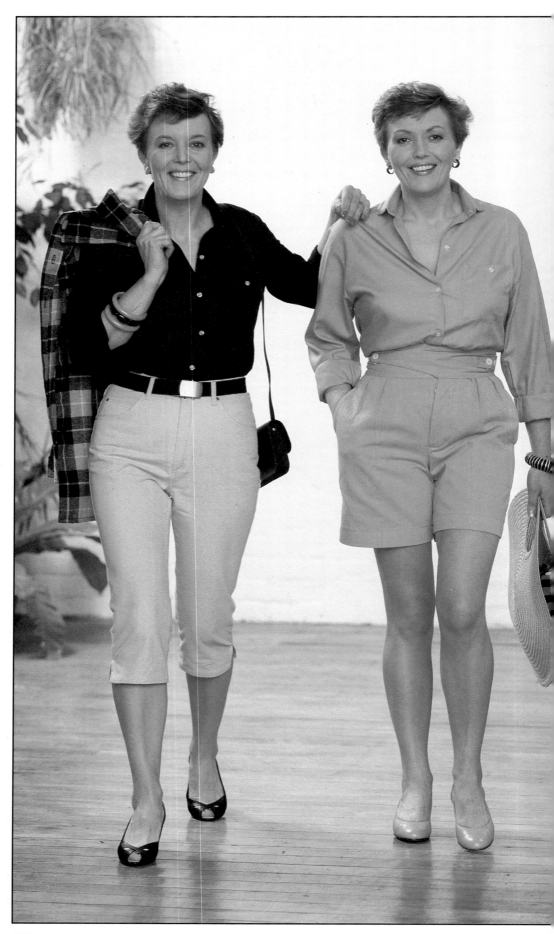

Mary and Julia's double success

Julia Colley had always believed she was meant to be 'Big Sister'. She was two years older than Mary and, at 1.68m (5ft 6in), 2cm (1 inch) taller. She put on 28.6kg (4½st) when she was expecting her first baby, but he accounted for less than 4.1kg (9lb) of it. Mary Levy at that time had no weight problems and, even when her two children were born, she somehow managed to stay around the 64kg (10st) mark. Mary badgered Julia to slim, but no diet seemed to work for long. Mary was always the one to suggest going out and about, especially in summer. She would sometimes try to get Julia to sunbathe in the garden but Julia preferred to stay indoors. Mary and Julia kept in touch by telephone most days and when Julia would ring with news of her latest diet, Mary would suggest she telephone when she had lost 1kg (2lb). But there was always some reason why Julia never managed to tackle her problem. It was as if she had settled for being fat but could not quite bring herself to admit it. It was only when Mary, to her great surprise, found herself gradually gaining more and more weight that they were able to help one another. Mary had to admit to Julia that she was finding it almost impossible to slim. Although mutual commiseration was good for their souls and soothed their tempers, it did little to improve their figures. They decided they needed someone to tell them where they had gone wrong; to give them a push and check on them until they could keep their weight under control. They had seen a local slimming club advertised and Mary went along as the advance party and reported back favourably to Julia. Julia joined the following week. What they were told made sense and they were given a thorough grounding in calorie values. Mary proposed that they walked to the club from home each week to burn up extra calories. In less than five months, the sisters were both stunning, attractive size-12s.

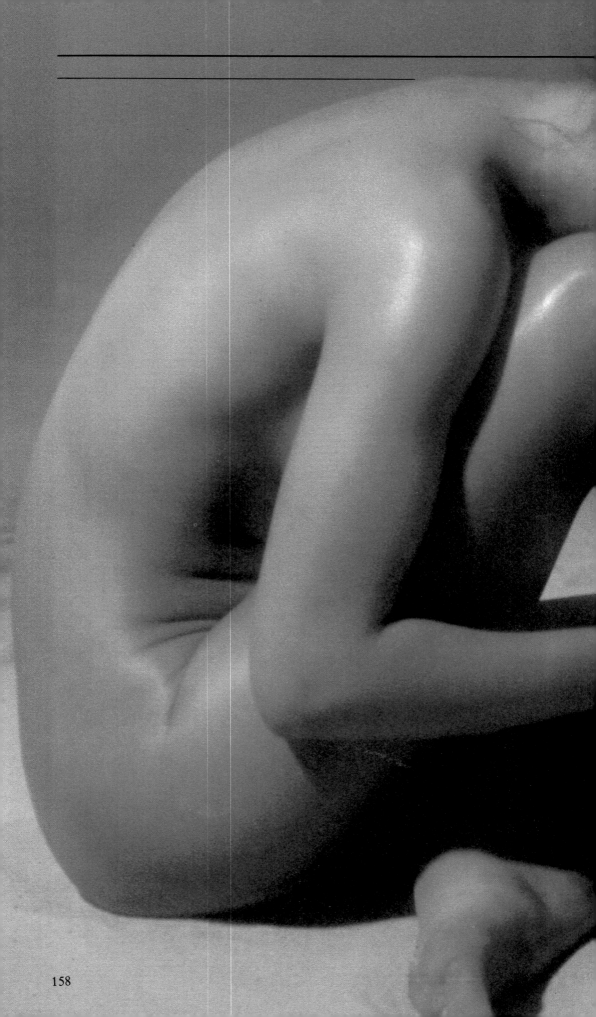

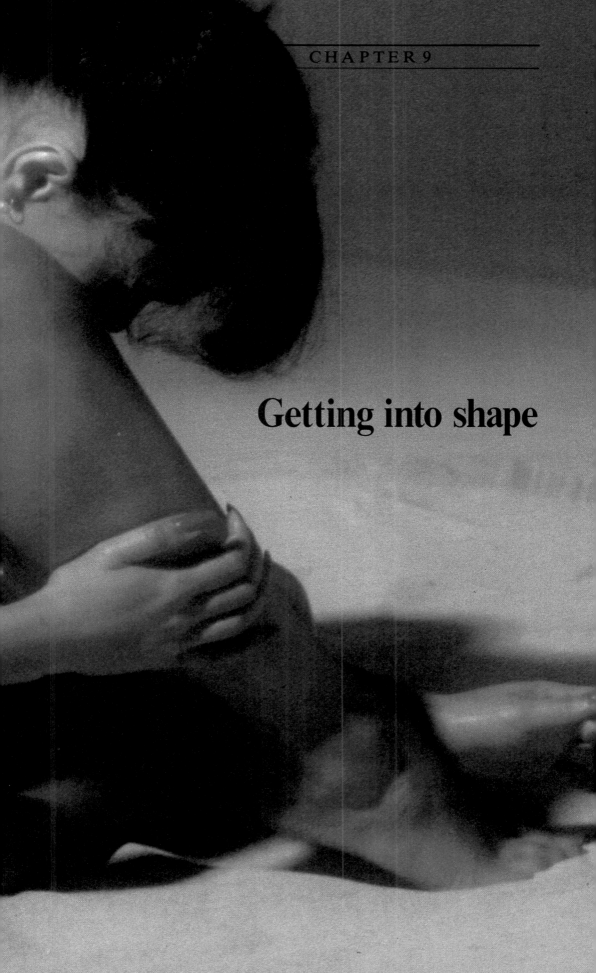

Getting into shape

Shaping up

Few women can say that they are totally satisfied with their body, whether they are young or old, plump or slim, or even top photographic models. It is not unusual to hear women bewailing their 'drooping pear shape', 'plump waistline' or 'flabby tummy'. As your slimming routine takes effect and you lose excess weight, you may find that your shape is not as streamlined as you would wish. For as fat disappears, flabby muscles show up and these can prevent you from looking nicely slim — just what you *do not* want when you have worked hard to get rid of unwanted weight.

One thing to remember is that fat seems to cling always in the places where you least want it. So if your waistline or your thighs are your biggest problem areas, you may have to get right down to your target weight before the final problem flab disappears. However, you can certainly trim your shape

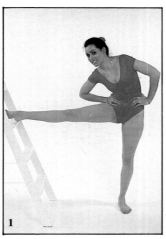

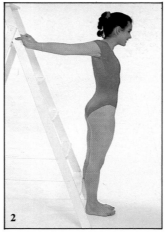

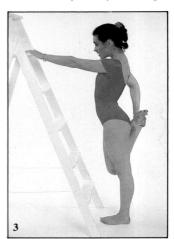

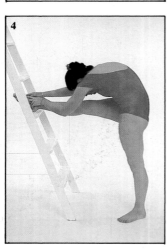

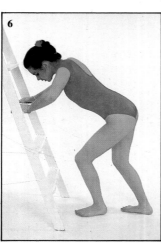

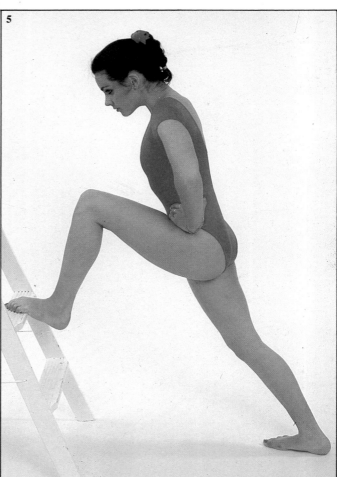

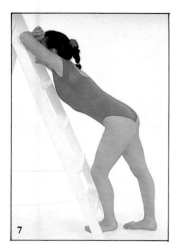

7

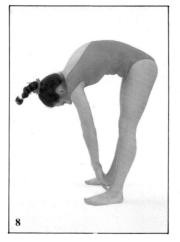

8

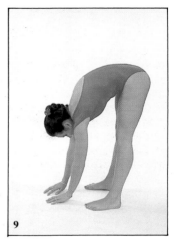

9

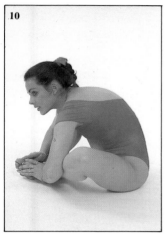

10

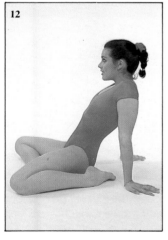

12

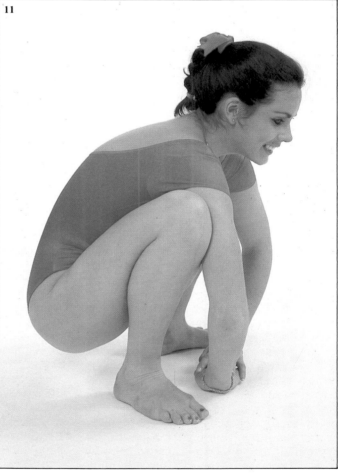

11

These stretching exercises will stretch your limbs and muscles before you embark on the shaping-up exercises.

1 Stand with one foot parallel to ground, and bend at waist towards it. Each leg for 15 seconds.

2 Holding the support with your hands behind you at shoulder level, straighten arms as you lean forwards. Hold your chin in and your chest up for 20 seconds.

3 Holding your right foot in your left hand, pull your heel towards buttocks. Hold 30 seconds.

4 Bend forwards from the waist until you feel the pull in your raised leg. Hold for 20 seconds, relax and repeat with other leg.

5 Hold your raised leg straight and bend your knee as your hips move forwards. Hold 30 seconds.

6 Keeping your back flat and heel down, lower hips as you bend knee. Hold 15 seconds.

7 Leaning on support, turn your hip inwards. Turn your hip sideways as you lean your shoulders in the opposite direction. Hold for 25 seconds for each hip.

8 & 9 With feet apart, bend forwards from hips bending knees. Straighten knees and hold for 15-25 seconds.

10 Feet together, hold your toes and bend forwards. Hold for 40 seconds.

11 From a standing position, squat down with your feet flat and toes pointed out at 15 degrees. Hold for 30 seconds.

12 With right leg bent and heel just outside right hip, bend left leg with left sole inside upper right leg. Hold for 30 seconds.

as you lose weight with exercises designed to tone up muscles that are not as firm as they should be. Take a look in your mirror and honestly assess where muscle sag shows — tummy, thighs, bottom, upper arms? Perhaps your bust droops or you have the faintest hint of a double chin?

The no-nonsense exercises in this chapter are tailored to attack muscles where they need chivvying most. You start on them gradually, working up to full measure as your body becomes more accustomed to the effort (if you have any worries about your health, consult your doctor first). To be really successful a certain amount of effort and determination will be needed on your part. The reward will be a much trimmer shape and a new confidence that you are looking your best.

Concentrate at first on your worst problem area rather than trying to do all the exercises. As you get into the habit of exercising for a few minutes every day you will probably find that it takes very little effort to incorporate some of the other exercises if you need them.

Before you embark on any other exercises, try this stretch which is an instant morale booster and also a treat for your back.

Stretch up slim

To lose several centimetres (inches) off your waist in seconds you simply need to start stretching your spine. There is nothing more instantly improving to any body.

Stand, with your feet just slightly apart, hands lightly clasped on top of your head; elbows back, shoulders down. Now try hard to push your crown up through your hands. Keeping that stretched spine upright, walk slowly about with a deliberate, high goose-stepping movement (or if you have not got room for that, just raise your knee high with each stride). Repeat this as often as possible.

Fix a motto in your mind for slim-stretch potential: *tail in, tum in, chin up!* Follow this advice and you can be sure that, whatever your weight, you are carrying it well. When you go out shopping, try to imagine that all your shopping is beautifully balanced on your head and walk tall.

Your newly stretched spine will give you an instantly slimmer look and stretching in this way gives a real mental lift.

Firming up

The following exercises are designed to tone up muscles rather than burn up lots of calories. We have suggested some high-calorie-burning exercises in the section entitled *Stepping up the calories you burn*.

You could incorporate a mixture of these exercises into your daily slimming programme. You may find that it is easiest to break your exercises into short sessions throughout the day — a muscle-toning exercise first thing in the morning before you dress, walking for half an hour at lunchtime to burn up extra calories and a second muscle-toning exercise in the evening before you go to bed. Try to establish a set routine so that exercising becomes a habit rather than a chore.

If your flab is due to the fact that you are still overweight, you must combine exercise with a diet to get satisfactory results. No form of exercise, however strenuous, will compensate for an excessive intake of food.

Firming up heavy thighs

Heavy thighs are not uncommon among many women who have otherwise good figures. They are, however, a problem that is shared by many women who have allowed themselves to become overweight. When they slim down, they may find that their thighs tend to remain big and flabby. For some women, too, the thigh is the area most vulnerable to weight gain. Whatever the cause, it is possible to trim down even massive thighs to a slim, firm shape by diet and our special thigh-reducing exercises. Continue to work at these to maintain firmness even after reducing flab in these areas. The best way to firm thighs is by using specific exercises which are designed to strengthen the weak muscles in this part of the leg. Firm flesh depends on firm muscles, and this can only come from hard work. Firming the thighs is always tough, especially at the beginning, and you must expect to experience some pain as muscles are tautened. If nothing hurts, you are being too easy with yourself!

Two warnings: if you are still very overweight, then please diet down until you are a reasonable size before starting this exercise plan; and because the movements are very strenuous, do not overdo them at first. Do each exercise two or three times for the first few days, then gradually increase the number until you can reach the maximum target.

How much improvement may you expect? There will be a gradual but very definite improvement from the start; but if you are over 40, it may take about a year before your thighs slim down and firm up to a good shape. If you are under 40, it will take less time, perhaps about six months or so.

If you do this routine every day, you can expect to see your thighs become more shapely within a few weeks. However, at this point you are likely to reach a plateau

CHAPTER 10

Staying slim

Once you have slimmed down
to the weight that suits
you best, how do you keep
it that way? If you have
clung to the fantasy
that *now* you can revert to
your 'normal' pattern of
carefree eating without
regaining any weight, forget it.
If that pattern was the
cause of your putting on
weight in the past, then
it will have the same
effect the second, third,
or even the fourth time
around. You have
got to find a new
way of eating.

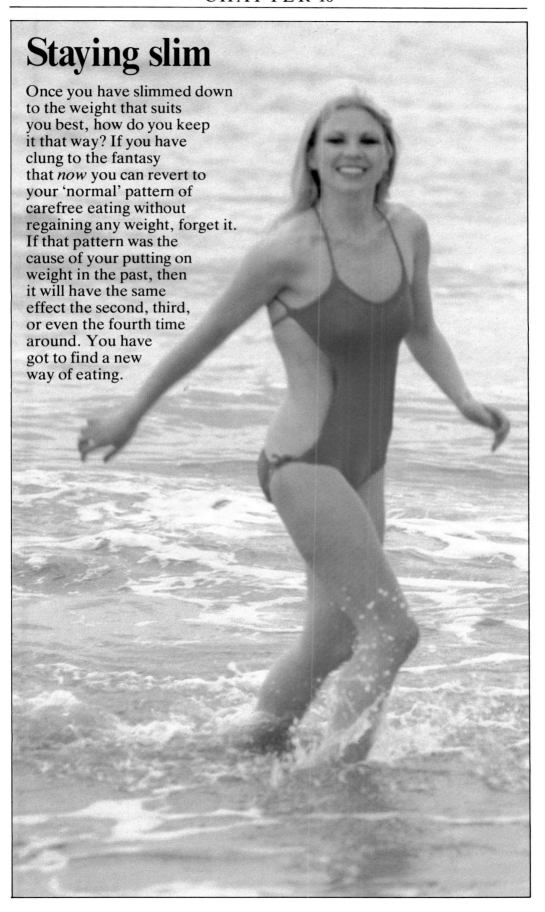

Slimmers who stay slim are rarely good all the time. They tend to balance out bad days with saintly ones. Here are four menus each totalling 300 calories — much too low a calorie total to diet on for a long period, but very effective as a one-day emergency measure.

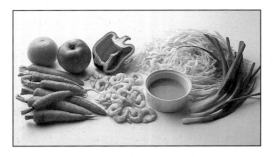

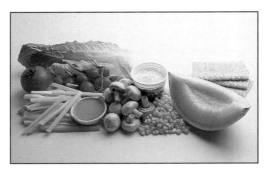

DAY 1

1 small orange
1 medium apple
250 (9oz) cabbage
225g (8oz) carrots
½ green pepper (capsicum)
3 spring onions or ½ medium onion
75g (3oz) peeled prawns
60ml (4 tablespoons) oil-free French dressing

Eat the pieces of fruit for breakfast or later in the day if you wish. The vegetables, prawns and dressing can be mixed together to make one big salad which you are free to dip into throughout the day.

DAY 3

300g (11oz) cantaloupe, honeydew or
  yellow melon, weighed with skin
50g (2oz) sweetcorn, cooked
75g (3oz) mushrooms
75g (3oz) radishes
3 sticks celery
50g (2oz) lettuce
30ml (2 tablespoons) oil-free French dressing
115g (4oz) cottage cheese, natural or with
  pineapple, peppers and onion
3 crispbreads
1 tomato

Start the day off with melon. Mix together the sweetcorn, mushrooms, radishes, celery and dressing and serve a good helping with lettuce for one meal; and the remainder with the cottage cheese, crispbreads and tomato for your second meal.

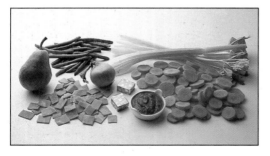

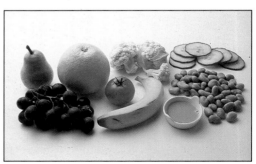

DAY 2

1 medium pear
3 medium carrots
50g (2oz) onion
50g (2oz) green beans
3 sticks celery
40g (1½oz) tomato purée
2 chicken stock cubes
50g (2oz) ham
850ml (1½ pint) water

The fruit can be eaten first thing or later. Chop vegetables and put in a pan with water, tomato purée and stock cubes. Bring to boil and simmer for 15 minutes. Discard any visible fat from ham, then chop lean and add to soup. Heat some soup for each meal.

DAY 4

1 medium grapefruit
175g (6oz) grapes
1 medium pear
1 small banana
150g (5oz) cauliflower
75g (3oz) broad beans, cooked
50g (2oz) cucumber
1 tomato
15ml (1 tablespoon) oil-free French dressing

You could sweeten grapefruit with a no-calorie artificial sweetener if you wish. Mix together the grapes, pear and banana for a fruit salad lunch; then chop and mix together the vegetables and toss with dressing for a main-meal salad.

How do they really stay trim?

The real experts on staying trim are those women who have succeeded in both their slimming and staying slim. You can learn from their example and advice.

'Quite frankly, as far as I'm concerned, eating is tied up with emotions. I find that when I am unhappy or emotionally a bit empty, I eat and eat; but when I am emotionally satisfied I just don't need stacks of food...' This comment came from a woman who was 12.7kg (2st) overweight all her life until she succeeded in solving her big weight problem. It crystallizes a major problem that many weight-prone women face by posing the question: can any normal human female eat in a restrained and weight-conscious way all the time? Many previously overweight women point to the relationship between eating and emotions.

A woman who had been overweight for 10 years, reaching more than 82.6kg (13st) at one time before getting her weight down to a slim 54.4kg (8st8lb), confessed that she has kept slim despite the fact that she still suffers from having a 'sweet tooth' and a couple of temptation days each month. She attributed these difficult days to pressures and tension rather than to a conscious craving for high-calorie foods. Another woman, who had become very slim after being moderately overweight for years, admitted to being an erratic eater, who found it relatively easy to stick to a moderate amount of food for a week or two but then dashed automatically to the biscuit tin whenever she was upset or harassed. These are women who have succeeded nevertheless in staying slim.

On that golden day when a woman finally achieves her goal and becomes slim at last, she will feel on top of the world. She may promise herself that *nothing* will ever induce her to become fat again, but how difficult is it for the average woman to keep to her resolve? Will she find that the desire to over-eat that made her fat has disappeared automatically with her surplus weight?

A recent survey asked a sample of successful slimmers whether, during the few months immediately following their dieting, they had found that they could not eat as much food as they had consumed before slimming. Only 18 per cent said that this was the case; the remaining slimmers said that their appetites were reduced, but only to a degree. They all agreed that it would have been very easy to slip back into eating the same pre-diet quantity of food if they had not made a conscious effort to discipline themselves. However, to a certain extent, most of them did stray occasionally from their new eating pattern.

Only 15 per cent succeeded in keeping their weight steady during the first few months. For the majority, the pattern was one of gaining a little weight and then of shedding weight again by more dieting.

During the early months of staying slim, it is more realistic to accept this slight fluctuation in weight level than to become guilt-obsessed by gaining even a little weight. The key factor lies in having a set weight of maybe 3kg (½st) over your ideal weight, above which you will *never* go.

Some women found at first that they gained 1½-2kg (3-4lb) every month, but then they would diet for a week to lose it all again. This did not prove difficult, as shedding 2kg (4lb) is simple after losing maybe 25kg (4st). Others experienced eating binges during which they would put weight on, and then diet for two weeks to take it off.

However, over the months, or even years in some cases, this habit of on-off dieting gradually merges into a more steady pattern of weight control, which rarely involves controlling food intake or choice of food on an unchanging, unerring everyday basis. Even a once-overweight woman who has succeeded in staying slim for 10 years can still admit to bad days when she finds it difficult to control her total food intake. However, these difficult days are balanced out by the good ones and as a result her weight stays fairly steady.

The majority of slimmers succeed in staying slim mainly by having learned about the calorie content of the foods they eat during dieting. This allows them to eat many of the foods they like without feeling guilty and to over-indulge a little on some days, notably at weekends, social occasions, or days when they are feeling pressurized and harassed. They know, however, that they can make up for these dietary lapses by choosing really low-calorie foods on other easier days.

Many women are 'weekday dieters' and 'weekend-indulgers'; thus they follow their routine of eating moderately during the week but eat large amounts of food when relaxing, socializing or entertaining at the weekend. In this way, they stay slim and their weight is relatively steady.

Other slimmers, who eat a lot at weekends, diet on Mondays and Tuesdays, and then eat moderately for the rest of the week. Thus they control their weight with the minimum of effort. They may think in terms of 14,000 calories per week rather than 2,000 calories a day. In this way, if their calorie intake is high on one day, they can eat foods that are lower in calories the next day. You may find that you grudge wasting calories on foods you can do without and prefer to enjoy your social life, eating and drinking what you like, and then eat low-calorie foods on your own during the week.

Research has shown that, although many

successful slimmers may slip back into a pattern of eating large quantities of food in the first few months following their dieting, those dieters who had kept slim for a longer period frequently reached a point when their appetite started to diminish and they needed less food than before.

Thirty-five per cent of the slimmers who were questioned in one survey said that they frequently left food on the plate because they felt too full to finish a large meal. These tended to be the women who had persevered in staying slim for long periods, and this evidence suggests that a form of automatic control may not set in until six months have elapsed after the end of the diet. However, some women experience immediate appetite reduction after dieting, while others are still tempted to eat over-large meals for a year or even more.

The majority of successful slimmers admit that, although they now eat less sugary and less starchy foods than when they were overweight, they still consume these foods but quite often in smaller amounts. These over-indulgences, however, make little or no difference to their weight, which remains steady. Although days of emotional distress, very often the pre-period days, are often the most dangerous for the most weight-prone women, a close runner-up is boredom. Most women discover that losing weight gives them the confidence to launch into a more active and sociable life and therefore there is less time to feel bored. Successful slimmers should be aware, however, that if they allow themselves to become inactive, uninterested or bored, they might easily resort to the eating habits that previously made them fat. Therefore, try to keep busy and active, especially by regular exercise. This will burn up your calorie output, firm up muscles and keep your figure trim while dispelling any boredom you might be feeling.

Perhaps the most important question that every slimmer will want to ask is whether the process of staying slim can ever become effortless? When this question was put to 100 women interviewed in a recent survey, 37 per cent replied that it was virtually effortless. The remainder, however, were still practising some degree of conscious self-control in a variety of ways, but usually the degree of effort decreased as time went on. Obviously, all these women considered the effort involved to be worthwhile or they would not make it. Talk to some successful slimmers and immediately you will be struck by the enthusiasm with which they describe the pleasures and compensations that had sustained their efforts to get slim and stay that way. They usually feel more confident,

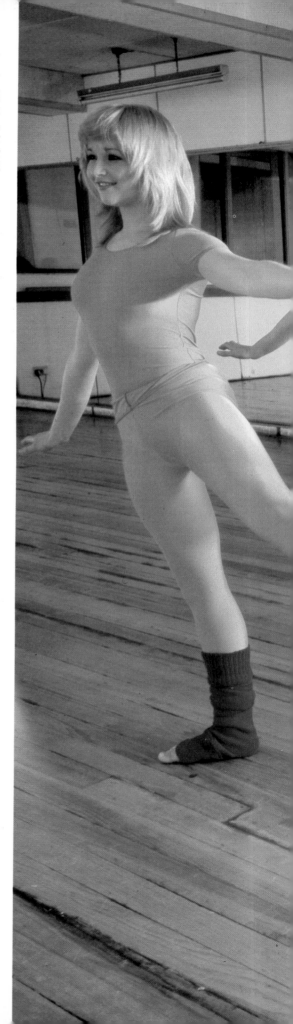

Chart of basic foods

Below you will find the calories, fibre and fat units in most basic foods. Where no figure is given, this means information on this food is presently unavailable. Some sweet foods and drinks do not contain fat but are still high in calories and could severely hamper your weight loss if you consume too much. We have, therefore, accorded them an equivalent fat unit count.

Abbreviations: C = calories; GF = grams fibre; FU = fat units; E = equivalent fat units

A	C	GF	FU
ALMONDS			
Shelled, per 28g/1oz	160	4.1	5.5
Ground,			
per 15ml/1 level tablespoon	40	1.0	1
per 20ml (Australian tablespoon)	50	1.3	1
Per almond, whole	10	0.2	0.5
Per sugared almond	15	0.2	0.5
ANCHOVIES			
Per 28g/1oz	40	0	1
Per anchovy fillet	5	0	0.25
ANCHOVY ESSENCE			
Per 5ml/1 level teaspoon	5	0	0
ANGELICA			
Per 28g/1oz	90	0	1E
Per average stick	10	0	0
APPLES			
Eating, per 28g/1oz, flesh only	13	0.6	0
Cooking, per 28g/1oz, fresh only	11	0.7	0
Medium whole eating, 142g/5oz	50	2.7	0
Medium whole cooking, 227g/8oz	80	4.3	0
Apple sauce, sweetened, per 15ml/			
1 level tablespoon	20	0	0
per 20ml (Australian tablespoon)	25	0	0
Apple sauce, unsweetened, per 15ml/			
1 level tablespoon	10	0.6	0
per 20ml (Australian tablespoon)	15	0.8	0
APRICOTS			
Canned in natural juice, per 28g/1oz	13	0.4	0
Canned in syrup, per 28g/1oz	30	0.4	0
Dried, per 28g/1oz	52	6.8	0.5
Fresh with stone, per 28g/1oz	7	0.5	0
Per dried apricot	10	1.3	0
ARROWROOT			
Per 28g/1oz	101	0.8	0
Per 5ml/level teaspoon	10	0	0
ARTICHOKES			
Globe, boiled, per 28g/1oz	4	0.7	0
Jerusalem, boiled, per 28g/1oz	5		0
ASPARAGUS			
Raw or boiled, soft tips, per 28g/1oz	5	0.4	0
Per asparagus spear	5	0.4	0
AUBERGINES (Eggplants)			
Raw, per 28g/1oz	4	0.7	0
Sliced, fried, 28g/1oz raw weight	60	0.7	2
Whole aubergine, 200g/7oz	28	5.0	0
Whole aubergine, sliced, fried, 200g/7oz			
raw weight	420	5.0	14
AVOCADO			
Flesh only, per 28g/1oz	63	0.6	2
Per half avocado, 105g/3¾oz	235	2.1	8.5

B	C	GF	FU
BACON (*see also gammon*)			
Per 28g/1oz			
Back rasher, raw	122	0	4
Collar joint, raw, lean and fat	91	0	3
Collar joint, boiled, lean only	54	0	1
Collar joint, boiled, lean and fat	92	0	2.5
Streaky rashers, raw	118	0	4
1 streaky rasher, well grilled or fried, 21g/¾oz raw weight	50	0	1
1 back rasher, well grilled or fried, 35g/ 1¼oz raw weight	80	0	1.5
1 bacon steak, well grilled, 100g/3½oz average raw weight	105	0	1.5
BAKING POWDER			
Per 28g/1oz	46	0	0
Per 5ml/1 level teaspoon	5	0	0
BAMBOO SHOOTS			
Canned, per 28g/1oz	5	0.1	0
BANANAS			
Small whole fruit, 115g/4oz	55	2.3	0
Medium whole fruit, 170g/6oz	80	3.4	0
Large whole fruit, 200g/7oz	95	4.0	0
BARCELONA NUTS			
Shelled, per 28g/1oz	181	2.9	6.5
BARLEY			
Pearl, raw, per 28g/1oz	102	1.8	0
Pearl, boiled, per 28g/1oz	34	0.6	0
Per 15ml/1 level tablespoon raw	45	0.8	0
Per 20ml (Australian tablespoon)	60	1.0	0
BASS			
Fillet, steamed, per 28g/1oz	35	0	0
BEAN SPROUTS			
Raw, per 28g/1oz	8	0.3	0
Boiled, per 28g/1oz	7	0.3	0
BEANS			
Per 28g/1oz			
Baked, canned in tomato sauce	20	2.1	0
Black eye beans, raw weight	93	7.2	0
Broad, boiled	30		
Butter, boiled	27	1.4	0
Butter, raw, dry weight	77	6.1	0
French, boiled	10	0.9	0
Haricot, boiled	26	2.1	0
Haricot, raw weight	77	7.2	0
Red kidney, canned	25	2.3	0
Red kidney, raw, dry weight	77	7.0	0
Mung, raw, dry weight	92	6.2	0
Runner, boiled	5	0.9	0
Runner, raw, green	7	0.9	0
Soya, dry weight	108	1.2	1.5
BEECH NUTS			
Shelled, per 28g/1oz	160		5
BEEF			
Per 28g/1oz			
Brisket, boiled, lean and fat	92	0	2.5
Brisket, raw, lean and fat	71	0	2
Ground beef, very lean, raw	45	0	0.5
Ground beef, very lean, fried and drained of fat	55	0	0.5
Ground beef, lean, fried and drained of fat, per 28g/1oz raw weight	40	0	0.5
Minced beef, raw	74	0	1.5
Minced beef, well fried and drained of fat	82	0	1
Minced beef, well fried and drained of fat per 28g/1oz raw weight	60	0	0.5

177

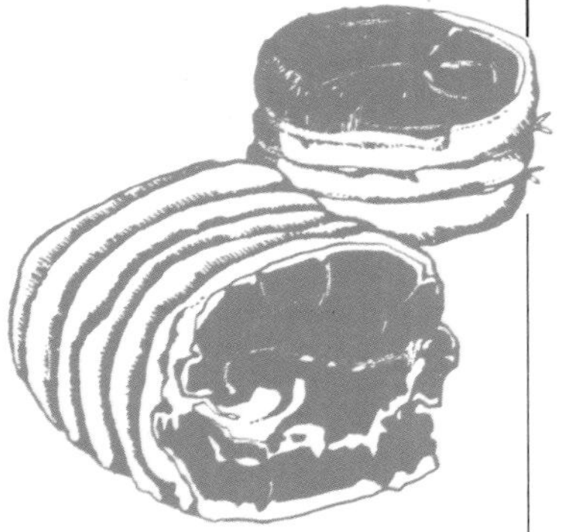

	C	GF	FU
Rump steak, fried, lean only	54	0	1
Rump steak, raw, lean and fat	56	0	1.5
Rump steak, grilled lean only, 28g/1oz	48	0	0.5
Rump steak, medium grilled, 170g/6oz raw	260	0	5.5
Rump steak, well grilled, 170g/6oz raw	290	0	4
Rump steak, rare grilled, 170g/6oz raw	310	0	6
Silverside, salted, boiled, lean and fat	69	0	1.5
Silverside, salted, boiled, lean only	49	0	0.5
Sirloin, roast, lean and fat	80	0	2
Sirloin, roast, lean only	55	0	1
Stewing steak, raw, lean only	35	0	0.5
Stewing steak, raw, lean and fat	50	0	1
Topside, raw, lean only	35	0	0.5
Topside, raw, lean and fat	51	0	1
Topside, roast, lean and fat	61	0	1
Topside, roast, lean only	44	0	0.5
BEEFBURGERS			
Beefburger, fresh or frozen, well grilled, 57g/2oz raw weight	115	0.2	3
Beefburger, fresh or frozen, grilled 113g/4oz raw weight	240	0.4	6
BEETROOT			
Raw, per 28g/1oz	8	0.9	0
Boiled, per 28g/1oz	12	0.7	0
Per baby beet, boiled	5	0.4	0
BILBERRIES			
Raw or frozen, per 28g/1oz	16		0
BISCUITS			
Per average biscuit			
Chocolate chip cookie	60		1.5
Digestive, large	70	0.8	0.5
Digestive, medium	55	0.6	0.5
Digestive, small	45	0.4	0.5
Fig roll	65	0.7	0.5
Garibaldi, per finger	30	0.3	0.5
Ginger nut	40	0.2	0.5
Ginger snap	35	0.2	0.5
Jaffa cake	50		0.5
Lincoln	40	0.1	0.5
Malted milk	40		0.5
Marie	30	0.2	0.25
Morning coffee	25	0.2	0.5
Nice	45		0.5
Osborne	35	0.2	0.25
Petit Beurre	30		0.5
Rich tea finger	25	0.2	0.25
Rich tea, round	45	0.2	0.5
Sponge finger	20	0.1	0.5
BLACKBERRIES			
Raw or frozen, 28g/1oz	8	2.5	0
Stewed, without sugar, per 28g/1oz	7	1.8	0
BLACKCURRANTS			
Raw or frozen, per 28g/1oz	8	2.5	0
Stewed without sugar, per 28g/1oz	7	2.1	0
BLOATERS			
Fillet, grilled, per 28g/1oz	71	0	1.5
On the bone, grilled per 28g/1oz	53	0	1.5
BRAINS			
Per 28g/1oz			
Calves' or lamb's, raw	31	0	1
Calves', boiled	43	0	1
Lamb's boiled	36	0	1
BRAN			
Per 28g/1oz	58	12.5	0.5
Per 15ml/level tablespoon	10	1.2	0
Per 20ml (Australian tablespoon)	15	1.6	0
BRAWN			
Per 28g/1oz	43	0	1.5

	C	GF	FU
BRAZIL NUTS			
Shelled, per 28g/1oz	175	2.5	6
Per nut, shelled	20	0.3	0.5
Per buttered brazil	40	0.3	0.5
Per chocolate brazil	55	0.3	0.5
BREAD			
Per 28g/1oz slice			
Black rye	90		0.5
Brown or wheatmeal	63	1.5	0.25
Currant	70	0.5	0.5
Enriched, eg. cholla	110	0.8	0.5
French	85	0.8	0.5
Fruit sesame	120		0.5
Granary	70		0.25
Light rye	70		0.25
Malt	70	1.4	0.5
Milk	80		0.5
Soda	75	0.65	0.25
Vogel	65		0.25
Wheatgerm, eg. Hovis and Vitbe	65	1.3	0.25
White	66	0.8	0.25
Wholemeal (100%)	61	2.4	0.25
Rolls, buns etc., each			
Baby bridge roll, 15g/½oz	35	0.4	0.25
Bagel, 42g/1½oz	150		1.5
Bap, 42g/1½oz	130	1.4	1.5
Bath bun, 42g/1½oz	120	1.1	0.5
Brioche roll, 45g/1¾oz	215		2
Chelsea bun, 90g/3¼oz	255	2.3	2.5
Croissant, 65g/2½oz	280		5.5
Crumpet, 42g/1½oz	75		0.5
Crusty roll, brown, 45g/1¾oz	145	2.9	0.5
Crusty roll, white, 45g/1¾oz	145	1.5	0.5
Currant bun, 45g/1¾oz	150	0.9	1.5
Devonshire split, with cream, 65g/2½oz	195		4
Dinner roll, soft, 42g/1½oz	130	1.2	0.5
Hot cross bun, 50g/2oz	180		1.5
Muffin, 60g/2¼oz	125		0.5
Pitta, 65g/2½oz	205		0.5
Scone, plain white, 50g/2oz	160	1.2	2
Soft brown roll, 45g/1¾oz	140	2.7	1
Soft white roll, 45g/1¾oz	150	1.4	1
Tea cake, 50g/2oz	155	1.2	1.5
Per 15ml/level tablespoon			
Breadcrumbs, dried	30	0.7	0
Breadcrumbs, white, fresh	8	0.1	0
Bread sauce	15	0.1	0.5
Per 20ml (Australian tablespoon)			
Breadcrumbs, dried	40	0.9	0
Breadcrumbs, white, fresh	10	0.1	0
Bread sauce	20	0.1	0.5
BREAKFAST CEREALS			
Per 28g/1oz			
All Bran cereal	70	8.0	0.25
Bran flakes	85	6.6	0
Cornflakes	100	0.5	0
Muesli or Swiss style	105	2.1	0.5
Porridge oats	115	4.2	0.5
Puffed wheat	100	4.3	0.25
Sultana bran	85	3.3	0
Weetabix or whole wheat biscuits, per biscuit	65	2.4	0.25
BROCCOLI			
Raw, per 28g/1oz	7	1.0	0
Boiled, per 28g/1oz	5	1.1	0
BRUSSELS SPROUTS			
Raw, per 28g/1oz	7	1.2	0
Boiled, per 28g/1oz	5	0.8	0
BUTTER			
All brands, per 28g/1oz	210	0	8

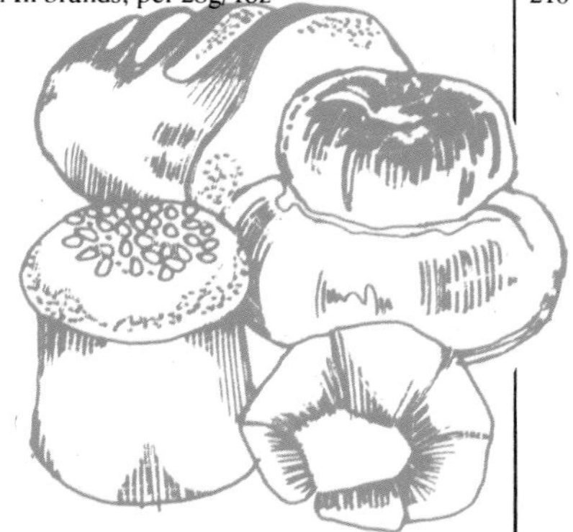

	C	GF	FU
CABBAGE			
Per 28g/1oz			
Raw	6	0.8	0
Boiled	4	0.7	0
Pickled red	3	0.9	0
CANDIED PEEL			
Per 28g/1oz	90	0	1
Per 15ml/level tablespoon	45	0	0.5
Per 20ml (Australian tablespoon)	60	0	0.5
CAPERS			
Per 28g/1oz	5		0
CARROTS			
Raw, per 28g/1oz	6	0.8	0
Boiled, per 28g/1oz	5	0.8	0
Per average carrot, 57g/2oz	12	1.6	0
CASHEW NUTS			
Shelled, per 28g/1oz	160	4.0	4
Per nut	15	0.3	0.5
CASSAVA			
Fresh, per 28g/1oz	43	0.3	0
CAULIFLOWER			
Raw, per 28g/1oz	4	0.6	0
Boiled, per 28g/1oz	3	0.5	0
CAVIAR			
Per 28g/1oz	75	0	1.5
CELERIAC			
Boiled, per 28g/1oz	4	1.4	0
CELERY			
Raw, per 28g/1oz	2	0.4	0
Boiled, per 28g/1oz	1	0.6	0
Per stick of celery	5	1.0	0
CHEESE			
Per 28g/1oz			
Austrian smoked	78	0	2.5
Babybel	97	0	2
Bavarian smoked	80	0	2
Bel Paese	96	0	3.5
Blue Stilton	131	0	4
Bonbel	102	0	3.5
Boursin	116	0	4
Bresse bleu	80	0	2
Brie	88	0	2.5
Caerphilly	120	0	3
Caithness Morven	110	0	3
Caithness full fat soft	110	0	3
Camembert	88	0	2.5
Cheddar	120	0	3.5
Cheese spread	80	0	2.5
Cheshire	110	0	3
Cheviot	120	0	3.5
Cotswold	105	0	3

	C	GF	FU
Cottage cheese, plain or with chives, onion, pepper or pineapple	27	0	0.5
Cream cheese	125	0	4.5
Curd cheese	54	0	1
Danbo	97	0	2.5
Danish Blue	100	0	3
Danish Elbo	97	0	2.5
Danish Esrom	90	0	2.5
Danish Fynbo	97	0	2.5
Danish Havarti	117	0	3.5
Danish Maribo	100	0	3
Danish Molbo	100	0	3
Danish Mozzarella	98	0	3
Danish Mycella	100	0	3
Danish Samsoe	101	0	3
Derby	110	0	3
Dolcellata	100	0	3
Double Gloucester	105	0	3
Edam	90	0	2.5
Emmenthal	115	0	3
Fetta	85	0	2.5
Gorgonzola	112	0	2.5
Gouda	100	0	3
Gruyère	117	0	3.5
Ilchester Cheddar and beer	112	0	3.5
Jarlsberg	95	0	2.5
Lancashire	109	0	3
Leicester	105	0	3
Norwegian blue	100	0	3
Norwegian Gjeost	133	0	4
Orangerulle	92	0	3
Orkney Claymore	111	0	3
Parmesan	118	0	3
Philadelphia	90	0	3.5
Port Salut	94	0	3
Processed	88	0	2.5
Rambol, with walnuts	117	0	3
Red Windsor	119	0	3.5
Riccotta	58	0	2
Roquefort	88	0	2
Sage Derby	115	0	3
Skimmed milk soft cheese (quark)	20	0	0.25
St Paulin	98	0	2.5
Tôme au raisin	94	0	2.5
Wensleydale	115	0	3
White Stilton	108	0	3
Per 15ml/level tablespoon			
Cottage cheese	15	0	0
Cream cheese	60	0	4.5
Curd cheese	25	0	1
Parmesan cheese	30	0	3
Per 20ml (Australian tablespoon)			
Cottage cheese	20	0	0
Cream cheese	75	0	6
Curd cheese	35	0	1
Parmesan cheese	40	0	4

CHERRIES	C	GF	FU
Fresh, with stones, per 28g/1oz	12	0.4	0
Glacé, per 28g/1oz	60		0
Per glacé cherry	10		0
CHESTNUTS			
Per 28g/1oz			
Shelled	48	1.9	0.5
With shells	40	1.6	0.25
Unsweetened chestnut purée	30		
CHICKEN			
Per 28g/1oz			
On bone, raw, no skin	25	0	0.25
Meat only, raw	34	0	0.5
Meat only, boiled	52	0	0.5
Meat only, roast	42	0	0.5
Meat and skin, roast	61	0	1.5
Chicken drumstick, raw, 100g/3½oz average raw weight	90	0	1.5
Chicken drumstick, grilled and skin removed, 100g/3½oz average weight	65	0	1
Chicken drumstick, grilled, 100g/3½oz raw weight	85	0	1.5
Chicken leg joint, raw 225g/8oz average weight, skin removed	410	0	2.5
Chicken leg joint, grilled and skin removed, 225g/8oz average weight	165	0	2
Chicken leg joint, grilled, with skin, 225g/8oz average weight	250	0	5
CHICORY			
Raw, per 28g/1oz	3	0.4	0
CHILLIES			
Dried, per 28g/1oz	85	7.1	0
CHIVES			
Per 28g/1oz	10		0
CHINESE LEAVES			
Raw, per 28g/1oz	7	0.6	0
CHOCOLATE			
Per 28g1/1oz			
Milk or plain	150	0	1.5
Cooking	155	0	1.5
Filled chocolates	130	0	1.5
Vermicelli	135	0	1.5
Per 5ml/level teaspoon			
Chocolate spread	20	0	0.25
Drinking chocolate	10	0	0
Vermicelli	20	0	0.25
CLAMS			
With shells, raw, per 28g/1oz	15	0	0
Without shells, raw, per 28g/1oz	25	0	
COB NUTS			
With shells, per 28g/1oz	39	0.6	1.5
Shelled, per 28g/1oz	108	1.7	3.5
Per nut	5	0	0
COCKLES			
Without shells, boiled, per 28g/1oz	14	0	0
COCOA POWDER			
Per 28g/1oz	88		2
Per 5ml/level teaspoon	10		0.5
COCONUT			
Per 28g/1oz			
Fresh	100	3.8	3.5
Desiccated	171	6.6	6
Fresh coconut milk, per 28ml/1floz	6	0	0
Creamed coconut	218		8
Desiccated, per 15ml/level tablespoon	30	1.1	1
Per 20ml (Australian tablespoon)	40	1.4	1
COD			
Per 28g/1oz			
Fillet, raw	22	0	0
Fillet, baked or grilled with a little fat	27	0	0.5
Fillet, poached in water or steamed	24	0	0
Frozen steaks, raw	19	0	0
On the bone, raw	15	0	0
COD LIVER OIL			
Per 5ml/teaspoon	40	0	1.5
COD ROE			
Raw, hard roe, per 28g/1oz	32	0	0.25
COFFEE			
Coffee beans, roasted and ground infusion	0	0	0
Instant, per 5ml/teaspoon	0	0	0
COLEY			
Per 28g/1oz			
Raw	21	0	0
On the bone, steamed	24	0	0
Fillet, steamed	28	0	0
COOKING OR SALAD OIL			
Per 28g/1oz	255	0	10

	C	GF	FU
Per 15ml/1 level tablespoon	120	0	5
Per 20ml (Australian tablespoon)	160	0	6
CORNED BEEF, CANNED			
Per 28g/1oz	62	0	1
CORNFLOUR			
Per 28g/1oz	100	0.8	0
Per 15ml/1 level tablespoon	33	0.3	0
Per 20ml (Australian tablespoon)	44	0.4	0
CORN OIL			
Per 28g/1oz	255	0	10
Per 15ml/1 level tablespoon	120	0	5
Per 20ml (Australian tablespoon)	160	0	6
CORN ON THE COB			
Average whole cob	155	4.5	0
COURGETTES (Zucchini)			
Raw per 28g/1oz	4	0.5	0
Per courgette, 65g/2½oz	10	1.3	0
CRAB			
With shell, per 28g/1oz boiled	7	0	0
Meat only, per 28g/1oz boiled	36	0	0.5
Average crab with shell	100	0	1.5
CRANBERRIES			
Per 28g/1oz	4	1.2	0
CRANBERRY SAUCE			
Per 28g/1oz	65		0.5E
Per 15ml/1 level tablespoon	45		0.5E
Per 20ml (Australian tablespoon)	60		0.5E
CREAM			
Per 28g/1oz			
Clotted	165	0	5.5
Double	127	0	5
Half cream	35	0	1
Imitation	85	0	3
Single	60	0	2
Soured	60	0	2
Sterilised, canned	65	0	2.5
Whipping	94	0	3.5
Per 15ml/1 level tablespoon			
Clotted	105	0	3.5
Double	55	0	2
Half cream	20	0	0.5
Imitation	55	0	2
Single	30	0	1
Soured	30	0	1
Sterilised, canned	35	0	1
Whipping	45	0	1.5
Per 20ml (Australian tablespoon)			
Clotted	140	0	4.5
Double	75	0	3
Half cream	25	0	0.5
Imitation	75	0	2.5
Single	40	0	1.5
Soured	40	0	1.5
Sterilised, canned	45	0	1.5
Whipping	60	0	2
CRISPS (potato)			
All flavours, per 28g/1oz	150	3.4	3.5
Lower fat, per 28g/1oz	125		2.5
CUCUMBER			
Raw, per 28g/1oz	3	0.1	0

CURRANTS	C	GF	FU
Per 28g/1oz	69	2.2	0.5E
Per 15ml/1 level tablespoon·	20	0.6	0.25
Per 20ml (Australian tablespoon)	28	0.9	0.25
CURRY PASTE OR CONCENTRATE			
Per 28g/1oz	40	0	1
CURRY POWDER			
Per 28g/1oz	66		0
Per 5ml/1 level teaspoon	12		0
CUSTARD APPLE			
Flesh only, per 28g/1oz	25		0
CUSTARD POWDER			
Per 28g/1oz	100	0.8	0
Per 15ml/1 level tablespoon	33	0.2	0
Per 20ml (Australian tablespoon)	44	0.3	0

D

DAMSONS	C	GF	FU
Fresh, with stones per 28g/1oz	11	1.0	0
Stewed, no sugar, per 28g/1oz	8	0.9	0
DATES			
Per 28g/1oz			
Dried, with stones	60	2.1	0.5
Dried, without stones	70	2.4	0.5
Fresh, with stones	30		0
Per date, fresh	15		0
DELICATESSEN SAUSAGES			
Per 28g/1oz			
Belgian liver sausage	90	0.1	2.5
Bierwurst	75	0	2.5
Bockwurst	180	0	5
Cervelat	140	0	4
Chorizo	140		3
Continental liver sausage	85	0.1	3
Frankfurter	80	0.3	2.5
French garlic sausage	90	0	3
Garlic sausage	70	0	2.5
Ham sausage	50	0	0.5
Kabanos	115	0	3.5
Krakowska	80	0	2.5
Liver sausage	88	0.1	2.5
Mettwurst	120		3.5
Mortadella, Italian	105	0	3
Polish country sausage	60		1
Polony	80	0.2	2
Pork boiling ring, coarse	110	0	3.5
Salami, Belgian	130	0	4
Salami, Danish	160	0	4.5
Salami, Hungarian	130	0	4
Salami, German	120	0	3.5
Saveloy	74	0.1	2
Smoked Dutch sausage	105	0	3
Smoked pork sausage	130	0	3.5
Smoked ham sausage	65	0	2
DRIPPING			
Per 28g/1oz	253	0	10
Per 15ml/1 level tablespoon	125	0	5
Per 20ml (Australian tablespoon)	165	0	6

DUCK	C	GF	FU
Per 28g/1oz			
Raw, meat only	35	0	0.5
Raw, meat, fat and skin	122	0	4.5
Roast, meat only	54	0	1
Roast, meat, fat and skin	96	0	3
DUCK EGGS			
100g/3½oz egg	170	0	4

E

EEL	C	GF	FU
Meat only, raw per 28g/1oz	48	0	1
Meat only, stewed in water, per 28g/1oz	57	0	1.5
Jellied eels plus some jelly, 85g/3oz	180	0	4
EGGS, each			
Size 1	95	0	2.5
Size 2	90	0	2.5
Size 3	80	0	2
Size 4	75	0	2
Size 5	70	0	2
Size 6	60	0	1.5
Yolk of size 3 egg	65	0	2
White of size 3 egg	15	0	0
EGG PLANTS			
see aubergines			
ENDIVE			
Raw, per 28g/1oz	3	0.6	0

F

FIGS	C	GF	FU
Dried, per 28g/1oz	60	5.2	0.5
Fresh, green, per 28g/1oz	12	0.7	0
Per dried fig	30	2.6	0.25
FLOUNDER			
On the bone, raw, per 28g/1oz	20	0	
On the bone, steamed, per 28g/1oz	15	0	
FLOUR			
Per 28g/1oz			
Buckwheat	99	0.3	0.25
Cassava	97	0.4	0
Granary	99		0
Maizemeal or Cornmeal (96%)	103	0.4	0.5
Maizemeal or Cornmeal (60%)	100	0.2	0
Potato	100	0.3	0
Rice	100	0.7	0
Rye (100%)	95	3.3	0.25
Soya, low fat	100	4.0	0.5
Soya, full fat	127	3.4	2.5
Wheatmeal	93	2.1	0.25
White, plain	99	1.0	0
White, self-raising	96	1.0	0
White, strong	96	0.8	0
Wholemeal	90	2.7	0.25
Yam	90	0.4	0

Per 15ml/1 level tablespoon	C	GF	FU
White	32	0.3	0
Wholemeal	29	0.9	0
Per 20ml (Australian tablespoon)			
White	43	0.4	0
Wholemeal	39	1.1	0
FRENCH DRESSING			
Per 15ml/tablespoon	75	0	3
Per 20ml (Australian tablespoon)	100	0	4
Oil-free, per 15ml/tablespoon	5	0	0
per 20ml (Australian tablespoon)	6	0	0
FRUIT			
Crystallised, per 28g/1oz	75	0	1E

G

GAMMON	C	GF	FU
Per 28g/1oz			
Gammon joint, raw, lean and fat	67	0	2
Gammon joint, boiled, lean and fat	76	0	2
Gammon joint, boiled, lean only	47	0	0.5
Gammon rashers, grilled, lean and fat	65	0	1
Gammon rashers, grilled, lean only	49	0	0.5
GARLIC			
One clove	0	0	0
GELATINE, powdered			
Per 15ml/1 level tablespoon	30	0	0
Per 28g/1oz	96	0	0
Per 20ml (Australian tablespoon)	40	0	0
Per 10g envelope	35	0	0
GHEE			
Per 28g/1oz	235	0	10
GHERKINS			
Per 28g/1oz	5		0
GINGER			
Ground, per 28g/1oz	73		0.5
Ground, 5ml/1 level teaspoon	8		0
Root, raw, peeled, 28g/1oz	18		0
Stem in syrup, strained, per 28g/1oz	60		0.5E
GOOSE			
Roast, on bone, per 28g/1oz	55	0	2
Roast, meat only (without skin), per 28g/1oz	90	0	2
GOOSEBERRIES			
Fresh, ripe dessert, per 28g/1oz	10	1	0
Fresh, cooking, per 28g/1oz	5	0.9	0
GRAPEFRUIT			
Per 28g/1oz			
Canned in syrup	17	0.2	0
Canned in natural juice	11	0.2	0
Flesh only	6	0.2	0
Flesh and skin	3	0.1	0
Juice, unsweetened, per 28ml/1floz	9	0.2	0
Juice, sweetened, per 28ml/1floz	11	0	0
Medium whole fruit, 340g/12oz	35	1.0	0
GRAPES			
Black, per 28g/1oz	14	0.1	0
White, per 28g/1oz	17	0.2	0

GREENGAGES	C	GF	FU
Fresh, with stones, per 28g/1oz	13	0.7	0
Stewed, with stones, no sugar, per 28g/1oz	11	0.6	0
GRENADINE SYRUP			
Per 28g/1oz	72	0	1E
GROUSE			
Roast, meat only, per 28g/1oz	50	0	0.5
GROUND RICE			
Per 28g/1oz	100	0.7	0
Per 15ml/1 level tablespoon	33	0.2	0
Per 20ml (Australian tablespoon)	44	0.3	0
GUAVAS			
Canned in natural juice, per 28g/1oz	12	1.0	0
GUINEA FOWL			
Roast, on bone, per 28g/1oz	30	0	0.5
Roast, meat only, per 28g/1oz	60	0	1

H

HADDOCK	C	GF	FU
Per 28g/1oz			
Fillet, raw	21	0	0
Fillet in breadcrumbs, fried	50	0.1	1
On the bone, raw	15	0	0
Smoked fillet, raw	25	0	0
HAGGIS			
Cooked, per 28g/1oz	88	0	2
HAKE			
Per 28g/1oz			
Fillet, raw	20	0	0
Fillet, steamed	30	0	0
Fillet, fried	60	0	1
On the bone, raw	10	0	0
HALIBUT			
Per 28g/1oz			
Fillet, steamed	37	0	0.25
On the bone, raw	26	0	0
On the bone, steamed	28	0	0
Steak, 170g/6oz	155	0	2
HAM			
Per 28g/1oz			
Chopped ham roll or loaf	75	0	1.5
Ham, boiled, lean	47	0	0.5
Ham, boiled, fatty	90	0	2
Honey roast ham	55	0	0.5
Old smokey ham	65	0	1
Maryland ham	55	0	0.25
Virginia ham	40	0	0.25
Ham steak, well grilled, 100g/3½oz, average raw weight	105	0	1
HARE			
Stewed, meat only per 28g/1oz raw	55	0	1
Stewed, on bone, per 28g/1oz	39	0	0.5
HASLET			
Per 28g/1oz	80	0	1.5
HAZELNUTS			
Shelled, per 28g/1oz	108	1.7	3.5
Per nut	5	0	0
Chocolate hazelnut whirl, each	40	0	0
HEART			
Per 28g/1oz			
Lamb's raw	34	0	0.5
Ox, raw	31	0	0.5
Pig's, raw	26	0	0.5

HERRING	C	GF	FU
Per 28g/1oz			
Fillet, raw	66	0	2
Fillet, grilled	56	0	1.5
On the bone, grilled	38	0	1
Rollmop herring	47	0	1
Rollmop herring, 70g/2½oz average weight	120	0	3
Whole herring, grilled, 128g/4½oz average weight	170	0	3.5
HERRING ROE			
Fried, per 28g/1oz	69	0	1.5
Raw, soft roe	23	0	0.5
HONEY			
Per 15ml/level tablespoon	60	0	0.5E
Per 20ml (Australian tablespoon)	80	0	1E
Per 5ml/1 teaspoon	20	0	0
HORSERADISH			
Fresh root, per 28g/1oz	17	2.4	0
Horseradish sauce, per 15ml/1 level tablespoon	13		0
per 20ml (Australian tablespoon)	17		0
HUMUS			
Per 28g/1oz	50		1.5

I

ICE-CREAM	C	GF	FU
Per 28g/1oz			
Chocolate	55	0	1.5
Coffee	50	0	1.5
Cornish dairy	50	0	1.5
Raspberry ripple	50	0	1.5
Soft ice-cream	45	0	1
Strawberry	50	0	1.5
Vanilla	45	0	1

J

JAM	C	GF	FU
Per 15ml/level tablespoon	45	0.2	0.5E
Per 5ml/level teaspoon	15	0	0
Per 20ml (Australian tablespoon)	60	0.2	0.5
JELLY			
Cubes as sold, per 28g/1oz	73	0	1E
Made up with water, per 142ml/¼ pint	85	0	1E
Per cube	30	0	0

K

KIDNEY	C	GF	FU
All types, raw, per 28g/1oz	25	0	0.25
Lamb's kidney, grilled, without fat, 57g/2oz average raw weight	50	0	0.5
KIPPERS			
Fillet, baked or grilled, without fat, per 28g/1oz	58	0	1
On the bone, baked, per 28g/1oz	31	0	0.5
Whole kipper, grilled, without fat, 170g/6oz	280	0	3.5

L

LAMB	C	GF	FU
Per 28g/1oz			
Breast, boned, raw, lean and fat	107	0	3.5
Breast, boned, roast, lean and fat	116	0	3.5
Breast, boned roast, lean only	71	0	1.5
Leg, raw, lean and fat, without bone	68	0	2
Leg, roast, lean and fat, without bone	75	0	2
Leg, roast, lean only, without bone	54	0	1
Scrag and neck, raw, lean and fat, weighed with bone	54	0	3
Scrag and neck, stewed, lean only, weighed with bone	38	0	1
Scrag and neck, stewed, lean only, weighed without bone	72	0	1.5
Shoulder, boned, roast, lean and fat	89	0	2.5
Shoulder, boned, roast, lean only	56	0	1
Chump chop, well grilled, 142g/5oz raw weight	205	0	6
Leg steak, boneless, well grilled, 225g/8oz raw weight	370	0	7
Loin chop, well grilled, 142g/5oz raw weight	175	0	6.5
LARD			
Per 28g/1oz	253	0	10
LAVERBREAD			
Per 28g/1oz	15	0.9	0.5
LEEKS			
Raw, per 28g/1oz	9	0.8	0
Average whole leek, raw	25	2.2	0
LEMON			
Flesh and skin, per 28g/1oz	4	1.5	0
Whole lemon, 142g/5oz	20	7.4	0
Lemon juice, per 15-20ml/1 tablespoon	0	0	0
LEMON CURD			
Per 28g/1oz	80	0	1E
LEMON SOLE			
Per 28g/1oz			
Fillet, steamed or poached	26	0	0
On the bone, raw	23	0	0
On the bone, steamed or poached	18	0	0
LENTILS			
Brown, raw, per 28g/1oz	104		0
Brown, boiled, per 28g/1oz	32		0
Red, raw, per 28g/1oz	86	3.3	0
Red, split, boiled, per 28g/1oz	28	1.0	0
Green, raw, per 28g/1oz	93		0
Green, boiled, per 28g/1oz	35		0
LETTUCE			
Fresh, per 28g/1oz	3	0.4	0
LIVER			
Per 28g/1oz			
Calves, raw	43	0	0.5

	C	GF	FU
Chicken's, raw	38	0	0.5
Chicken's, fried	55	0	1
Lamb's, raw	51	0	1
Lamb's, fried	66	0	1.5
Ox, raw	46	0	1
Pig's, raw	44	0	0.5
LOBSTER			
With shell, boiled, per 28g/1oz	12	0	0.25
Meat only, boiled, per 28g/1oz	34	0	0.5
LOGANBERRIES			
Fresh, per 28g/1oz	5	1.8	0
Canned in natural juice, per 28g/1oz	15	1	0
LOW-FAT SPREAD			
All brands, per 28g/1oz	105	0	4
Per 5ml/level teaspoon	15	0	0.5
LUNCHEON MEAT			
Per 28g/1oz	89	0	2.5

M

	C	GF	FU
MACARONI			
Per 28g/1oz			
White, raw	105	0.8	0.25
Wholewheat, raw	95	2.8	0.25
White, boiled	33	0.3	0
Wholewheat, boiled	34	0.9	0
MACEDONIA NUTS			
Per 28g/1oz	188	0.7	6.5
MACKEREL			
Per 28g/1oz			
Fillet, raw	63	0	1.5
Kippered mackerel	62	0	1.5
Smoked mackerel fillet	70	0	2.5
Whole raw mackerel, 225g/8oz	320	0	7.5
MAIZE			
Whole grain, per 28g/1oz	103	0.6	0.5
MANDARINS			
Canned in natural juice, per 28g/1oz	11	0.1	0
Fresh, weighed with skin, per 28g/1oz	7	0.4	0
Medium whole fruit, 75g/3oz	20	0.9	0
MANGO			
Raw, per 28g/1oz	17	0.4	0
Canned in syrup, per 28g/1oz	22	0.3	0
Mango chutney, per 15ml/1 level tablespoon	40	0.3	0
per 20ml (Australian tablespoon)	55	0.4	0
MAPLE SYRUP			
Per 15ml/tablespoon	50	0	0.5E
MARGARINE			
All brands including those labelled 'high in polyunsaturates', per 28g/1oz	210	0	8
MARMALADE			
Per 28g/1oz	74	0.2	1.0E
Per 15ml/1 level tablespoon	45	0.1	0.5E
Per 20ml (Australian tablespoon)	60	0.1	0.5E
MARRON GLACE			
Per 28g/1oz	74	0	1
MARROW			
Raw, flesh only, per 28g/1oz	5	0.5	0
Boiled, per 28g/1oz	2	0.2	0

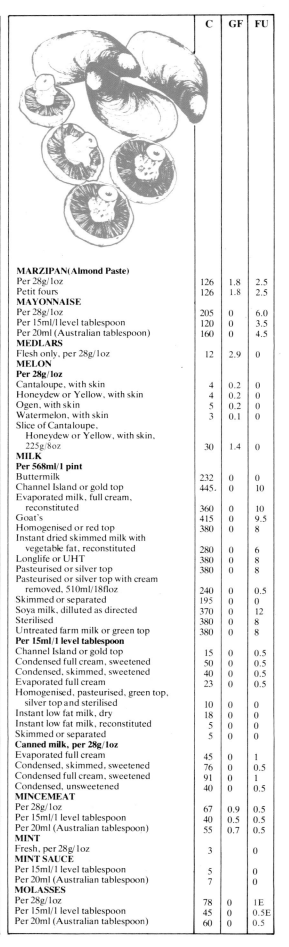

	C	GF	FU
MARZIPAN(Almond Paste)			
Per 28g/1oz	126	1.8	2.5
Petit fours	126	1.8	2.5
MAYONNAISE			
Per 28g/1oz	205	0	6.0
Per 15ml/1 level tablespoon	120	0	3.5
Per 20ml (Australian tablespoon)	160	0	4.5
MEDLARS			
Flesh only, per 28g/1oz	12	2.9	0
MELON			
Per 28g/1oz			
Cantaloupe, with skin	4	0.2	0
Honeydew or Yellow, with skin	4	0.2	0
Ogen, with skin	5	0.2	0
Watermelon, with skin	3	0.1	0
Slice of Cantaloupe, Honeydew or Yellow, with skin, 225g/8oz	30	1.4	0
MILK			
Per 568ml/1 pint			
Buttermilk	232	0	0
Channel Island or gold top	445	0	10
Evaporated milk, full cream, reconstituted	360	0	10
Goat's	415	0	9.5
Homogenised or red top	380	0	8
Instant dried skimmed milk with vegetable fat, reconstituted	280	0	6
Longlife or UHT	380	0	8
Pasteurised or silver top	380	0	8
Pasteurised or silver top with cream removed, 510ml/18floz	240	0	0.5
Skimmed or separated	195	0	0
Soya milk, diluted as directed	370	0	12
Sterilised	380	0	8
Untreated farm milk or green top	380	0	8
Per 15ml/1 level tablespoon			
Channel Island or gold top	15	0	0.5
Condensed full cream, sweetened	50	0	0.5
Condensed, skimmed, sweetened	40	0	0.5
Evaporated full cream	23	0	0.5
Homogenised, pasteurised, green top, silver top and sterilised	10	0	0
Instant low fat milk, dry	18	0	0
Instant low fat milk, reconstituted	5	0	0
Skimmed or separated	5	0	0
Canned milk, per 28g/1oz			
Evaporated full cream	45	0	1
Condensed, skimmed, sweetened	76	0	0.5
Condensed full cream, sweetened	91	0	1
Condensed, unsweetened	40	0	0.5
MINCEMEAT			
Per 28g/1oz	67	0.9	0.5
Per 15ml/1 level tablespoon	40	0.5	0.5
Per 20ml (Australian tablespoon)	55	0.7	0.5
MINT			
Fresh, per 28g/1oz	3		0
MINT SAUCE			
Per 15ml/1 level tablespoon	5		0
Per 20ml (Australian tablespoon)	7		0
MOLASSES			
Per 28g/1oz	78	0	1E
Per 15ml/1 level tablespoon	45	0	0.5E
Per 20ml (Australian tablespoon)	60	0	0.5

	C	GF	FU
MUESLI			
Per 28g/1oz	105	2.1	0.5
Per 15ml/1 level tablespoon	30	0.5	0
Per 20ml (Australian tablespoon)	40	0.7	0
MULBERRIES			
Raw, per 28g/1oz	10	0.4	0
MULLET			
Raw, flesh only, per 28g/1oz	40	0	0.5
MUSHROOMS			
Raw, per 28g/1oz	4	0.7	0
Sliced and fried, per 28g/1oz	60	1.1	2
MUSSELS			
With shells, boiled, per 28g/1oz	7	0	0
Without shells, boiled, per 28g/1oz	25	0	0.25
Per mussel	10	0	0
MUSTARD AND CRESS			
Raw, per 28g/1oz	3	1	0
Whole carton	5	1.6	0
MUSTARD			
Dry, per 28g/1oz	128		0
Made mustard, English, per 5ml/1 level teaspoon	10		0

	C	GF	FU
NECTARINES			
Whole fruit, medium	50	2.5	0
NOODLES			
Cooked, per 28g/1oz	33	0.5	0
NUTMEG			
Powdered, per 2.5ml/½ level teaspoon	0	0	0

	C	GF	FU
OATMEAL			
Raw, per 28g/1oz	114	2	1
Per 15ml/1 level tablespoon, raw	40	0.7	0.5
Per 20ml (Australian tablespoon), raw	55	0.8	0.5
OCTOPUS			
Raw, per 28g/1oz	20	0	0
OKRA (ladies' fingers)			
Raw, per 28g/1oz	5	0.9	0

	C	GF	FU
OLIVE OIL			
Per 28ml/1floz	255	0	10
Per 15ml/1 level tablespoon	120	0	5
OLIVES			
Stoned, in brine, per 28g/1oz	29	1.2	1
With stones, in brine, per 28g/1oz	23	1	1
Per stuffed olive	5	0.2	0
ONIONS			
Per 28g/1oz			
Raw	7	0.4	0
Boiled	4	0.3	0
Fried, sliced	98	1.3	3.5
Dried, per 15ml/1 level tablespoon	10	0.6	0
Whole onion, raw, 85g/3oz	20	1.2	0
Pickled onion, each	5	0.2	0
Cocktail onion, each	1	0	0
ORANGES			
Flesh only, per 28g/1oz	10	0.6	0
Flesh with skin, per 28g/1oz	7	0.4	0
Whole fruit, small, 142g/5oz	35	2.1	0
Whole fruit, medium, 225g/8oz	60	3.4	0
Whole fruit, large, 284g/10oz	75	4.2	0
ORANGE JUICE			
Per 28ml/1floz			
Canned, sweetened	15	0	0.5E
Unsweetened	11	0	0
OXTAIL			
Stewed, without bone, per 28g/1oz	69	0	1.5
On the bone, stewed and skimmed of fat, per 28g/1oz	26	0	0.5
OYSTERS			
With shells, raw, per 28g/1oz	2	0	0
Without shells, raw, per 28g/1oz	14	0	0
Per oyster	5	0	0

	C	GF	FU
PARSLEY			
Fresh, per 28g/1oz	6	2.6	0
Parsley sauce, per 15ml/1 level tablespoon	45	0	0.5
per 20ml (Australian tablespoon)	60	0	0.5
PARSNIPS			
Per 28g/1oz			
Raw	14	1.1	0
Boiled	16	0.7	0
Roast	30		0.5
PARTRIDGE			
Roast, on bone, per 28g/1oz	36	0	0.5
Roast, meat only, per 28g/1oz	60	0	0.5
PASSION FRUIT			
Flesh only, per 28g/1oz	10	4.5	0
PASTA			
White, all shapes, raw, per 28g/1oz	105	0.8	0.25
White, boiled, per 28g/1oz	33	0.3	0
Wholewheat, raw	95	2.8	0.25
Wholewheat, boiled	34	0.9	0
PASTRY			
Per 28g/1oz			
Choux, raw	60	0.2	1.5
Choux, baked	95	0.4	2
Flaky, raw	120	0.4	3
Flaky, baked	160	0.6	4
Shortcrust, raw	130	0.6	3
Shortcrust, baked	150	0.7	3
PAW PAW (Papaya)			
Canned in syrup, per 28g/1oz	18	0.1	0.25E
Fresh, flesh only, per 28g/1oz	11	0.2	0
PEACHES			
Canned in natural juice, per 28g/1oz	13	0.2	0
Canned in syrup, per 28g/1oz	25	0.2	0.25
Fresh, with stones, per 28g/1oz	9	0.3	0
Whole fruit, 113g/4oz	35	1.4	0
PEANUTS			
Per 28g/1oz			
Shelled, fresh	162	2.3	5
Dry roasted	160	2.3	5

	C	GF	FU
Roasted and salted	162	2.3	5
Peanut butter	177	2.1	5.5
Per peanut	5	0	0
PEARS			
Per 28g/1oz			
Cooking pears, raw, peeled	10	0.8	0
Dessert pears	8	0.5	0
Canned in syrup	22	0.5	0.25
Whole fruit, medium, 142g/5oz	40	2.4	0
PEAS			
Per 28g/1oz			
Frozen	15	2.2	0
Canned, garden	13	1.8	0
Canned, processed	23	2.2	0
Dried, raw	81	4.7	0
Dried, boiled	29	1.4	0
Split, raw	88	3.4	0
Split, boiled	33	1.4	0
Per 30ml/1 rounded tablespoon			
Dried, boiled	30	1.3	0
Fresh, boiled	10	1.1	0
Pease pudding	35		0
Per 40ml (Australian rounded tablespoon)			
Dried, boiled	40	1.8	0
Frozen, boiled	13	1.1	0
Pease pudding	45		0
PECANS			
Per nut	15	0	1
PEPPER			
Powdered, per pinch	0	0	0
PEPPERS (capsicums)			
Red or green, per 28g/1oz	4	0.3	0
Average pepper, 142g/5oz	20	1.4	0
PERCH			
White, raw, per 28g/1oz	35	0	0.5
Yellow, raw, per 28g/1oz	25	0	0.5
PHEASANT			
Meat only, roast, per 28g/1oz	60	0	1
On the bone, roast, per 28g/1oz	38	0	0.5
PICKLES AND RELISHES			
Mixed pickles, per 28g/1oz	5	0.5	0
Per 15ml/1 level tablespoon			
Piccalilli	15	0.3	0
Ploughmans	35	0.3	0
Sweet pickle	35	0.3	0
Per 20ml (Australian tablespoon)			
Piccalilli	20	0.4	0
Ploughmans	45	0.4	0
Sweet pickle	45	0.4	0
PIGEON			
Meat only, roast, per 28g/1oz	65	0	1.5
On the bone, roast, per 28g/1oz	29	0	0.5
PIKE			
Raw fillet, per 28g/1oz	25	0	0
PILCHARDS			
Canned in tomato sauce, per 28g/1oz	36	0	0.5
PIMENTOS			
Canned in brine, per 28g/1oz	6	0.2	0

	C	GF	FU
PINEAPPLES			
Canned in natural juice, weighed with juice, per 28g/1oz	15	0.3	0
Canned in syrup, per 28g/1oz	22	0.3	0.25
Fresh, weighed without skin and core, per 28g/1oz	13		
Ring of canned, drained pineapple in syrup	35	0.4	0.25E
Ring of canned, drained pineapple in natural juice	20	0.4	0
PISTACHIO NUTS			
Shelled, per 28g/1oz	180	0.5	**5.5**
Per nut	5		0
PLAICE			
Fillet, raw or steamed	26	0	0.25
Fillet, in batter, fried	79	0.2	2
Fillet, in breadcrumbs, fried	65	0.1	1.5
PLANTAIN			
Per 28g/1oz			
Green, raw	32	1.6	0
Green, boiled	35	1.8	0
Ripe, fried	76	1.6	1
PLUMS			
Per 28g/1oz			
Cooking plums with stones, stewed without sugar	6	0.6	0
Fresh dessert plums, with stones	10	0.6	0
Cooking plums, with stones	7	0.7	0
Victoria dessert plum, medium, each	15	0.9	0
POLLACK			
On the bone, raw, per 28g/1oz	25	0	0
POLONY			
On the bone, raw, per 28g/1oz	80	0.2	2
POMEGRANATE			
Flesh only, per 28g/1oz	20		0
Whole pomegranate, 205g/7¼oz	65		0
POPCORN			
Per 28g/1oz	110	0.3	1
PORK			
Per 28g/1oz			
Belly rashers, raw, lean and fat	108	0	3.5
Belly rashers, grilled, lean and fat	113	0	3.5
Fillet, raw, lean only	42	0	1
Leg, raw, lean and fat, weighed without bone	76	0	2.5
Leg, raw, lean only, weighed without bone	42	0	1
Leg, roast, lean and fat	81	0	2
Leg, roast, lean only	52	0	0.5
Crackling	190	0	4

Left column	C	GF	FU
Scratchings	185	0	4
Pork chop, well grilled, 184g/6½oz raw weight, fat removed	240	0	4
POTATOES			
Per 28g/1oz			
Raw	25	0.6	0
Old, baked, weighed with skin	24	0.7	0
Boiled, old potatoes	23	0.3	0
Boiled, new potatoes	22	0.6	0
Canned, new potatoes drained	15	0.7	0
Chips (average thickness)	70	0.6	7.5
Crisps	150	3.4	3.5
Roast, large chunks	40	0.6	0.5
Sauté	40	0.6	0.5
Instant mashed potato powder, per 15ml/level tablespoon, dry	40	1.0	0
Per 20ml (Australian tablespoon)	55	0.3	0
Jacket-baked potato, 200g/7oz raw weight	170	5	0
PRAWNS			
With shells, per 28g/1oz	12	0	0
Without shells, per 28g/1oz	30	0	0.25
Per shelled prawn	2	0	0
PRUNES			
Per 28g/1oz			
Dried, no stones	46	4.6	0.5E
Stewed, without sugar, fruit and juice without stones	21	2.1	0
Prune juice	25	0	0
Per prune	10	0	0
PUMPKIN			
Raw, flesh only per 28g/1oz	4	0.1	0

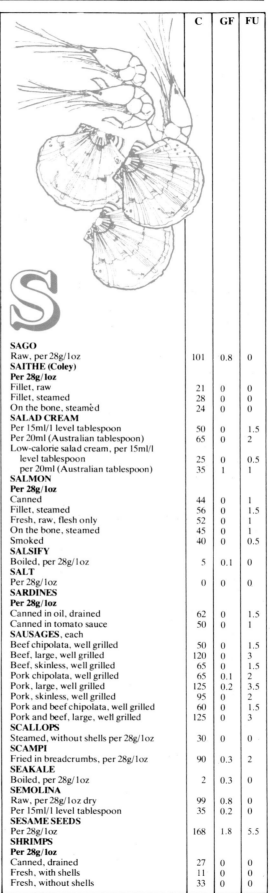

	C	GF	FU
QUINCES			
Raw, per 28g/1oz	7	1.8	0
RABBIT			
Per 28g/1oz			
Meat only, raw	35	0	0.5
Meat only, stewed	51	0	1.5
On the bone, stewed	26	0	0.5
RADISHES			
Fresh, per 28g/1oz	4	0.5	0
Per radish	2	0.2	0
RAISINS			
Dried, per 28g/1oz	70	1.9	1E
Per 15ml/1 level tablespoon	25	0.7	0.25E
Per 20ml (Australian tablespoon)	35	0.9	0.25E
RASPBERRIES			
Fresh or frozen, per 28g/1oz	7	2.1	0
Canned in syrup, drained, per 28g/1oz	25	1.4	0.25E
REDCURRANTS			
Fresh, per 28g/1oz	6	2.3	0
Redcurrant jelly, per 5ml/1 level teaspoon	15		0
RHUBARB			
Raw, per 28g/1oz	2	0.7	0
Stewed without sugar, per 28g/1oz	2	0.6	0
RICE			
Per 28g/1oz			
Brown, raw	99	1.2	0.25
White, raw	102	0.3	0
White, boiled	35	0.1	0
Brown, boiled	33	0.4	0
ROCK			
Seaside rock, per 28g/1oz	95	0	1E

Right column	C	GF	FU
SAGO			
Raw, per 28g/1oz	101	0.8	0
SAITHE (Coley)			
Per 28g/1oz			
Fillet, raw	21	0	0
Fillet, steamed	28	0	0
On the bone, steamed	24	0	0
SALAD CREAM			
Per 15ml/1 level tablespoon	50	0	1.5
Per 20ml (Australian tablespoon)	65	0	2
Low-calorie salad cream, per 15ml/1 level tablespoon	25	0	0.5
per 20ml (Australian tablespoon)	35	1	1
SALMON			
Per 28g/1oz			
Canned	44	0	1
Fillet, steamed	56	0	1.5
Fresh, raw, flesh only	52	0	1
On the bone, steamed	45	0	1
Smoked	40	0	0.5
SALSIFY			
Boiled, per 28g/1oz	5	0.1	0
SALT			
Per 28g/1oz	0	0	0
SARDINES			
Per 28g/1oz			
Canned in oil, drained	62	0	1.5
Canned in tomato sauce	50	0	1
SAUSAGES, each			
Beef chipolata, well grilled	50	0	1.5
Beef, large, well grilled	120	0	3
Beef, skinless, well grilled	65	0	1.5
Pork chipolata, well grilled	65	0.1	2
Pork, large, well grilled	125	0.2	3.5
Pork, skinless, well grilled	95	0	2
Pork and beef chipolata, well grilled	60	0	1.5
Pork and beef, large, well grilled	125	0	3
SCALLOPS			
Steamed, without shells per 28g/1oz	30	0	0
SCAMPI			
Fried in breadcrumbs, per 28g/1oz	90	0.3	2
SEAKALE			
Boiled, per 28g/1oz	2	0.3	0
SEMOLINA			
Raw, per 28g/1oz dry	99	0.8	0
Per 15ml/1 level tablespoon	35	0.2	0
SESAME SEEDS			
Per 28g/1oz	168	1.8	5.5
SHRIMPS			
Per 28g/1oz			
Canned, drained	27	0	0
Fresh, with shells	11	0	0
Fresh, without shells	33	0	0

SKATE	C	GF	FU
Fillet, in batter, fried, per 28g/1oz	57	0.1	1
SMELTS			
Without bones, fried, per 28g/1oz	115	0	1
SNAILS			
Flesh only, per 28g/1oz	25	0	0
SOLE			
Per 28g/1oz			
Fillet, raw	23	0	0
Fillet, steamed or poached	26	0	0
On the bone, steamed or poached	18	0	0
SPAGHETTI			
Per 28g/1oz			
White, raw	105	0.8	0.25
Wholewheat, raw	95	2.8	0.25
White, boiled	33	0.3	0
Wholewheat, boiled	30	0.9	0
Canned in tomato sauce	17	0.1	0
SPINACH			
Boiled, per 28g/1oz	9	1.7	0
SPRATS			
Fried without heads, per 28g/1oz	110	0	4
SPRING GREENS			
Boiled, per 28g/1oz	3	1.1	0
SPRING ONIONS (scallions)			
Raw, per 28g/1oz	10	0.4	0
Per onion	3	0.1	0
SQUID			
Flesh only, raw per 28g/1oz	25	0	0
STRAWBERRIES			
Fresh or frozen, per 28g/1oz	7	0.6	0
Canned, drained, per 28g/1oz	23		0
Per fresh strawberry	2	0.1	0
STURGEON			
On the bone, raw, per 28g/1oz	25	0	0
SUET			
Shredded, per 28g/1oz	235	0	8.5
Per 15ml/1 level tablespoon	85	0	3
Per 20ml (Australian tablespoon)	115	0	4
SUGAR			
White, brown, caster, Demerara, granulated, icing, per 28g/1oz	112	0	1E
Per 15ml/1 level tablespoon	50	0	0.5E
Per 20ml (Australian tablespoon)	70	0	0.5E
SULTANAS			
Dried, per 28g/1oz	71	1.9	0.5
Per 15ml/1 level tablespoon	25	0.7	0.25
Per 20ml (Australian tablespoon)	35	0.9	0.25
SUNFLOWER SEED OIL			
Per 28g/1oz	255	0	10
Per 15ml/1 tablespoon	120	0	5
Per 20ml (Australian tablespoon)	160	0	6
SWEDES			
Raw, per 28g/1oz	6	0.7	0
Boiled, per 28g/1oz	5	0.8	0
SWEETBREADS			
Lamb's, raw, per 28g/1oz	37	0	1
SWEETCORN			
Canned in brine, per 28g 1oz	22	1.6	0
Fresh, kernels only, boiled, per 28g/1oz	25	1.3	0
Frozen, per 28g/1oz	25	1.3	0
Whole medium cob	155	4.5	0

SWEETS	C	GF	FU
Per 28g/1oz			
Barley sugar	100	0	1
Boiled sweets	93	0	1
Butterscotch	115	0	1
Filled chocolates	130		1.5
Fudge	111	0	1.5
Liquorice allsorts	105		1
Marshmallows	90	0	1
Nougat	110		1
Nut brittle or crunch	120		1
Peppermints	110	0	1
Toffees	122		1

TANGERINES	C	GF	FU
Flesh only, per 28g/1oz	10	0.5	0
Flesh with skin, per 28g/1oz	7	0.4	0
Whole fruit, 75g/3oz	20	1.2	0
TAPIOCA			
Dry per 28g/1oz	102	0.8	0
TARAMASALATA			
Per 28g/1oz	135	0	5
TARTARE SAUCE			
Per 15ml/1 level tablespoon	35		1
Per 20ml (Australian tablespoon)	45		1
TEA			
All brands, per cup, no milk	0	0	0
TOMATOES			
Per 28g, 1oz			
Raw	4	0.4	0
Canned	3	0.2	0
Fried, halved	20	0.8	0.5
Fried, sliced	30	0.8	0.5
Ketchup	28	0	0
Purée	19	0	0
Whole medium tomato, 57g/2oz	8	0.8	0
Per 15ml/1 level tablespoon			
Chutney	45	0.3	0
Ketchup	15		0
Purée	10		0
Per 20ml (Australian tablespoon)			
Chutney	60	0.4	0
Ketchup	20		0
Purée	13		0
TONGUE			
Per 28g/1oz			
Lamb's, raw	55	0	1.5
Lamb's, lean only, stewed	82	0	2.5
Ox, lean only, boiled	83	0	2.5
TREACLE			
Black, per 28g/1oz	73	0	1
Per 15ml/1 level tablespoon	50	0	0.5
Per 20ml (Australian tablespoon)	65	0	0.5
TRIPE			
Dressed, per 28g/1oz	17	0	0.25
Stewed, per 28g/1oz	28	0	0.5

TROUT	C	GF	FU
Fillet, smoked, per 28g/1oz	38	0	0.5
Whole trout, poached or grilled without fat, 170g/6oz	150	0	2
Whole smoked trout, 156g/5½oz	150	0	2
TUNA			
Per 28g/1oz			
Canned in brine, drained	30	0	0
Canned in oil	82	0	2
Canned in oil, drained	60	0	1.5
TURKEY			
Per 28g/1oz			
Meat only, raw	30	0	0.25
Meat only, roast	40	0	0.25
Meat and skin, roast	48	0	0.5
TURNIPS			
Raw, per 28g/1oz	6	0.8	0
Boiled, per 28g/1oz	4	0.6	0

V

VEAL	C	GF	FU
Per 28g/1oz			
Fillet, raw	31	0	0.25
Fillet, roast	65	0	1
Jellied veal, canned	35	0	0
VENISON			
Roast meat only, per 28g/1oz	56	0	0.5
VINEGAR			
Per 28ml/1floz	1	0	0

W

WALNUTS	C	GF	FU
Shelled, per 28g/1oz	149	1.5	5
Per walnut half	15	0.1	0.5
WATERCHESTNUTS			
Per 28g/1oz	10	0.2	0
WATERCRESS			
Per 28g/1oz	4	0.9	0
WATERMELON			
Flesh only, per 28g/1oz	6	0.3	0
Flesh with skin, per 285g/10oz slice	30	0.8	0

WHEATGERM	C	GF	FU
Per 28g/1oz	100	0.6	1
Per 15ml/1 level tablespoon	18	0.1	0.25
Per 20ml (Australian tablespoon)	24	0.1	0.25
WHELKS			
With shells, boiled, per 28g/1oz	4	0	0
Without shells, boiled, per 28g/1oz	26	0	0
WHITEBAIT			
Fried coated in flour, per 28g/1oz	149	0	5
WHITE PUDDING			
As sold, per 28g/1oz	128	0	3
WHITING			
Per 28g/1oz			
Fillet, fried	54	0	1
Fillet, steamed	26	0	0.25
On the bone, fried in breadcrumbs	49	0	1
On the bone, steamed	18	0	0.25
WINKLES			
With shells, boiled, per 28g/1oz	4	0	0
Without shells, boiled, per 28g/1oz	21	0	0
WORCESTERSHIRE SAUCE			
Per 28ml/1floz	20	0	0
Per 15ml/1 level tablespoon	13	0	0
Per 20ml (Australian tablespoon)	17	0	0

Y

YAMS	C	GF	FU
Raw, per 28g/1oz	37	1.2	0
Boiled, per 28g/1oz	34	1.1	0
YEAST			
Fresh, per 28g/1oz	15	1.9	0
Dried, per 28g/1oz	48	6.1	0
Dried, per 5ml/1 level teaspoon	8	1.0	0
YOGHURT			
Per 150g/5oz carton			
Low fat, natural	75	0	0.5
Low fat, flavoured	115	0	0.5
Low fat, fruit	135	0	0.5
Low fat, nut	150	2.5	1.5
YORKSHIRE PUDDING			
Cooked, per 28g/1oz	60	0.3	1

Index

Numbers in *italics* refer to illustrations

Index of recipes

Picture Credits
All-Sport Photographic: page 36
Martin Brigdale: page 133
Tim Chadsey: pages 107, 113
Laurie Evans: page 125
Chris Knaggs: pages 97, 103, 105, 109, 111, 115, 119, 121, 123, 127, 129, 131, 135, 137
Spectrum Colour Library: pages 34, 40
Susan Griggs Agency: pages 58, 142–3, 170–1
Vital Magazine: pages 29, 30, 31, 33, 35, 41, 42, 43, 47, 158–9, 160–1
Graham Young: pages 99, 101, 117
Cover: Gary Compton